OXFORD SPECIALIST HANDBOOKS
IN CARDIOLOGY

Paediatric Cardiology

T0295117

Oxford Specialist Handbooks published and forthcoming

Oxford Specialist Handbooks In Cardiology

Paediatric Cardiology

FIRST EDITION

EDITED BY

Thomas Day

Honorary Consultant Paediatric and Fetal Cardiologist, Evelina London Children's Hospital, Guy's and St Thomas' NHS Foundation Trust, London, UK; Research Fellow, School of Biomedical Engineering and Imaging Sciences, King's College London, UK

Aaron Bell

Consultant Paediatric Cardiologist, Evelina London Children's Hospital, Guy's and St Thomas' NHS Foundation Trust, London, UK

Sadia Quyam

Consultant in Paediatric Cardiology and Pulmonary Hypertension, Great Ormond Street Hospital for Children, London, UK

John Simpson

Professor of Paediatric and Fetal Cardiology, Evelina London Children's Hospital, Guy's and St Thomas' NHS Foundation Trust, London, UK

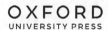

OXFORD
UNIVERSITY PRESS

OXFORD
UNIVERSITY PRESS

Great Clarendon Street, Oxford, OX2 6DP,
United Kingdom

Oxford University Press is a department of the University of Oxford.
It furthers the University's objective of excellence in research, scholarship,
and education by publishing worldwide. Oxford is a registered trade mark of
Oxford University Press in the UK and in certain other countries

© Oxford University Press 2024

The moral rights of the authors have been asserted

First Edition published in 2024

Published in the United States of America by Oxford University Press
198 Madison Avenue, New York, NY 10016, United States of America

British Library Cataloguing in Publication Data
Data available

Library of Congress Control Number: 2023952609

ISBN 978-0-19-886390-8

DOI: 10.1093/med/9780198863908.001.0001

Printed in the UK by
Ashford Colour Press Ltd, Gosport, Hampshire

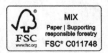

Contents

Contents

Contributors

Dr Tazeen Ashraf

Consultant in Clinical Genetics,
Great Ormond Street Hospital for
Children NHS Foundation Trust,
London, UK
*Chapter 8: Genetics and paediatric
cardiology*

Dr Aaron Bell

Consultant Paediatric Cardiologist,
Evelina London Children's Hospital,
Guy's and St Thomas' NHS
Foundation Trust,
London, UK
*Chapter 2: Evaluation of clinical
presentations*
*Chapter 3: Structural congenital heart
disease*

Dr Hannah Bellsham-Revell

Consultant in Paediatric Cardiology,
Evelina London Children's Hospital,
Guy's and St Thomas NHS
Foundation Trust,
London, UK
*Chapter 3: Structural congenital heart
disease*

Dr Sophie Bertaud

Consultant in Paediatric Palliative
Medicine,
Great Ormond Street Hospital for
Children NHS Foundation Trust,
London, UK
Chapter 17: Paediatric palliative care

Dr Gianfranco Butera

Department of Cardiology,
Cardiac Surgery and Heart Lung
Transplantation,
ERN GUARD HEART: Bambino
Gesù Hospital and Research Institute
IRCCS,
Rome, Italy
*Chapter 7: Cardiac catheterization
and intervention*

Dr Elena Cervi

Consultant Cardiologist,
Centre for Inherited Cardiovascular
Diseases,
Great Ormond Street Hospital for
Children NHS Foundation Trust,
London, UK
*Chapter 8: Genetics and paediatric
cardiology*

Dr Thomas Day

Honorary Consultant Paediatric and
Fetal Cardiologist, Evelina London
Children's Hospital,
Guy's and St Thomas' NHS
Foundation Trust,
London, UK;
Research Fellow, School of
Biomedical Engineering and Imaging
Sciences, King's College
London, UK
*Chapter 3: Structural congenital heart
disease*
*Chapter 11: Heart muscle disease and
cardiac transplantation*
*Chapter 15: Commonly used drugs in
paediatric cardiology*
*Chapter 18: Urgent care and
emergencies*

Dr Matthew Fenton

Consultant Paediatric Cardiologist,
Great Ormond Street Hospital for
Children NHS Foundation Trust,
London, UK
*Chapter 11: Heart muscle disease and
cardiac transplantation*

Dr Alessandra Frigiola

Consultant Cardiologist,
ACHD Specialist
Guy's and St Thomas NHS
Foundation Trust,
Honorary Senior Clinical Lecturer,
King's College,
London, UK
*Chapter 14: Transition and adult
congenital heart disease*

Dr Nicola Gregg
Highly Specialist Clinical Psychologist,
Evelina London Children's Hospital,
Guy's and St Thomas NHS
Foundation Trust,
London, UK
*Chapter 16: Promoting psychological
adjustment and well-being*

Dr Jennifer Handforth
Consultant in Paediatric Infectious
Disease,
Evelina London Children's Hospital,
Guy's and St Thomas NHS
Foundation Trust,
London, UK
Chapter 13: Multisystem disorders

Dr David F A Lloyd
Consultant in Paediatric and Fetal
Cardiology,
Evelina London Children's Hospital,
Guy's and St Thomas NHS
Foundation Trust,
London, UK;
Senior Research Fellow,
King's College,
London, UK
*Chapter 3: Structural congenital heart
disease*
*Chapter 18: Urgent care and
emergencies*

Dr Owen Miller
Consultant in Paediatric and Fetal
Cardiology, Evelina London
Children's Hospital,
Guy's and St Thomas NHS
Foundation Trust,
London, UK
Chapter 13: Multisystem disorders

Dr Gabrielle Norrish
Academic Clinical Lecturer,
Great Ormond Street Hospital for
Children NHS Foundation Trust,
Institute of Cardiovascular Science,
University College,
London, UK
*Chapter 11: Heart muscle disease and
cardiac transplantation*

Dr Kuberan Pushparajah
Consultant in Paediatric Cardiology,
Clinical Lead for Paediatric and
Congenital Cardiac MRI,
Evelina London Children's
Hospital,
Guy's and St Thomas NHS
Foundation Trust,
London, UK
*Chapter 4: Cardiac investigations in
children*

Dr Sadia Quyam
Consultant in Paediatric Cardiology
and Pulmonary Hypertension,
Great Ormond Street Hospital for
Children,
London, UK
*Chapter 4: Cardiac investigations in
children*
Chapter 5: Cardiac surgery
*Chapter 7: Cardiac catheterization
and intervention*
*Chapter 12: Paediatric pulmonary
hypertension*

Dr Will Regan
Consultant in Paediatric Cardiology
and Electrophysiology,
Evelina London Children's Hospital,
Guy's and St Thomas NHS
Foundation Trust,
London, UK
*Chapter 4: Cardiac investigations in
children*
*Chapter 7: Cardiac catheterization
and intervention*
Chapter 10: Paediatric arrhythmia

Prof Eric Rosenthal
Consultant Paediatric and Adult
Congenital Cardiologist,
Evelina London Children's Hospital,
Guy's and St Thomas NHS
Foundation Trust,
London, UK
*Chapter 4: Cardiac investigations in
children*
*Chapter 7: Cardiac catheterization
and intervention*
Chapter 10: Paediatric arrhythmia

# # #

I

Mr. Caner Salih
Chief of Congenital Cardiac Surgery,
Children's Cardiorespiratory and
Intensive Care,
Evelina London Clinical Group,
Guy's and St Thomas NHS
Foundation Trust,
London, UK
Chapter 5: Cardiac surgery

Prof Gurleen Sharland
Consultant in Fetal Cardiology,
Evelina London Children's Hospital,
Guy's and St Thomas' NHS Trust,
London, UK
Chapter 9: Fetal cardiology

Dr Jacob Simmonds
Consultant in Paediatric Cardiology
and Co-Director of Cardiothoracic
Transplantation,
Department of Paediatric
Cardiology,
Great Ormond Street Hospital for
Children NHS Foundation Trust,
London, UK
*Chapter 11: Heart muscle disease and
cardiac transplantation*

Prof John Simpson
Professor of Paediatric and Fetal
Cardiology,
Evelina London Children's Hospital,
Guy's and St Thomas' NHS
Foundation Trust,
London, UK
*Chapter 3: Structural congenital heart
disease*
*Chapter 4: Cardiac investigations in
children*
*Chapter 6: The single-ventricle
circulation*
Chapter 9: Fetal cardiology
Chapter 13: Multisystem disorders

Dr Paraskevi Theocharis
Consultant in Paediatric Cardiology,
Evelina London Children's Hospital,
Guys and St Thomas NHS
Foundation Trust,
London, UK
*Chapter 4: Cardiac investigations in
children*
*Chapter 11: Heart muscle disease and
cardiac transplantation*
Chapter 13: Multisystem disorders

Dr Trisha V. Vigneswaran
Clinical Lead for Fetal Cardiology,
Consultant in Fetal and Paediatric
Cardiology, Evelina London
Children's Hospital,
Guys and St Thomas NHS Foundation
Trust,
London, UK
*Chapter 3: Structural congenital heart
disease*

Dr James Wong
Consultant in Paediatric Cardiology,
Evelina London Children's Hospital,
Guy's and St Thomas NHS
Foundation Trust,
London, UK
*Chapter 3: Structural congenital heart
disease*
*Chapter 4: Cardiac investigations in
children*

Prof Vita Zidere
Consultant in Paediatric and Fetal
Cardiology,
Evelina London Children's Hospital,
Guy's and St Thomas' NHS Trust,
London, UK
Chapter 1: Cardiac morphology
*Chapter 3: Structural congenital heart
disease*

Dr Dan Taylor
Consultant Anaesthetist,
Evelina London Children's Hospital,
Guy's and St Thomas' NHS Trust,
London, UK
Chapter 5: Cardiac surgery

Dr Matthew Jones
Consultant Congenital Cardiologist,
Evelina London Children's Hospital,
Guys and St Thomas NHS
Foundation Trust,
London, UK
*Chapter 7: Cardiac catheterization
and intervention*

Dr Federica Brancato
Department of Woman and
Child Health, Policlinico Gemelli
Universitary Foundation IRCCS,
Catholic University of Sacre Hearth
Sacred Heart,
Rome, Italy
*Chapter 7: Cardiac catheterization
and intervention*

Dr Shahin Moledina
Consultant Paediatric Cardiologist,
Great Ormond Street Hospital for
Children NHS Foundation Trust,
London, UK
*Chapter 12: Paediatric pulmonary
hypertension*

Prof Sahar Mansour
Consultant and Honorary Professor
in Clinical Genetics,
St George's University Hospital
NHS Trust,
London, UK
*Chapter 8: Genetics and paediatric
cardiology*

Symbols and abbreviations

>	greater than		CHARGE	Coloboma, heart defects, choanal Atresia, growth Retardation/Renal abnormalities, Genital abnormalities, Ear anomalies
≥	greater than or equal to			
<	less than			
≤	less than or equal to			
±	with/without			
2D	two-dimensional		CHD	congenital heart disease
3D	three-dimensional		cMRI	cardiac magnetic resonance imaging
ACE	angiotensin-converting enzyme			
ACEi	angiotensin-converting enzyme inhibitor(s)		CNS	clinical nurse specialist
			CO	cardiac output
ACHD	adult congenital heart disease		CO_2	carbon dioxide
ACS	acute coronary syndromes		CPB	cardiopulmonary bypass
AF	atrial fibrillation		CPET	cardiopulmonary exercise testing
ALCAPA	anomalous origin of the left coronary artery from the pulmonary artery		CPVT	catecholaminergic ventricular tachycardia
AP	anteroposterior		CT	computed tomography
ARF	acute rheumatic fever		CVP	central venous pressure
ARVC	arrhythmogenic right ventricular cardiomyopathy		CXR	chest X-ray
			DC	direct current
AS	aortic stenosis		DCM	dilated cardiomyopathy
ASD	atrial septal defect		DKS	Damus–Kaye–Stansel
AT	anaerobic threshold		DORV	double-outlet right ventricle
AV	atrioventricular		ECG	electrocardiogram/electrocardiography
AVN	atrioventricular node			
AVNRT	atrioventricular nodal re-entry tachycardia		ECMO	extracorporeal membrane oxygenation
AVRT	atrioventricular re-entry tachycardia		ENT	ear, nose, and throat
			ES	Eisenmenger syndrome
AVSD	atrioventricular septal defect		FBC	full blood count
BAS	balloon atrial septostomy		FiO_2	fraction of inspired oxygen
BPD	bronchopulmonary dysplasia		GA	general anaesthetic
BTT	Blalock–Thomas–Taussig		GAS	group A Streptococcus
ccTGA	congenitally corrected transposition of the great arteries		GP	general practitioner
			Hb	haemoglobin
			HCM	hypertrophic cardiomyopathy
			HTN	hypertension

ICD	implantable cardioverter defibrillator	PO_2	partial pressure of oxygen
IE	infectious endocarditis	POTS	postural orthostatic tachycardia syndrome
IPAH	idiopathic pulmonary arterial hypertension	PPHN	persistent pulmonary hypertension of the newborn
IUD	intrauterine device	PS	pulmonary stenosis
IV	intravenous	PV	pulmonary vein
IVC	inferior vena cava	PVR	pulmonary vascular resistance
IVIG	intravenous immunoglobulin	QF-PCR	quantitative fluorescence polymerase chain reaction
KD	Kawasaki disease	Qp	pulmonary blood flow
LA	left atrium	Qs	systemic blood flow
LBBB	left bundle branch block	QTc	corrected QT interval
LFT	liver function test	RA	right atrium
LQTS	long QT syndrome	RBBB	right bundle branch block
LV	left ventricle	RCM	restrictive cardiomyopathy
LVEDP	left ventricular end-diastolic pressure	RHD	rheumatic heart disease
		RV	right ventricle
LVOT	left ventricular outflow tract	RVH	right ventricular hypertrophy
LVOTO	left ventricular outflow tract obstruction	RVOT	right ventricular outflow tract
		RVOTO	right ventricular outflow tract obstruction
MAPCA	major aortopulmonary collateral artery	SCD	sudden cardiac death
MDT	multidisciplinary team	SVC	superior vena cava
MPA	main pulmonary artery	SVR	systemic vascular resistance
mPAP	mean pulmonary artery pressure	SVT	supraventricular tachycardia
NBM	nil by mouth	TAPVD	total anomalous pulmonary venous drainage
NSAID	non-steroidal anti-inflammatory drug	TGA	transposition of the great arteries
O_2	oxygen	TNF	tumour necrosis factor
PA	pulmonary artery	TOE	transoesophageal echocardiography
PAH	pulmonary arterial hypertension	TPG	transpulmonary gradient
PaO_2	partial pressure of oxygen in the arterial blood	TTE	transthoracic echocardiogram/ echocardiography
PAP	pulmonary artery pressure	U&E	urea and electrolytes
PAPVD	partial anomalous pulmonary venous drainage	VA	ventriculoarterial
PCO_2	partial pressure of carbon dioxide	VACTERL	Vertebral defects, Anal atresia, Cardiac defects, Tracheo-oEsophageal fistula, Renal anomalies, Limb abnormalities
PCWP	pulmonary capillary wedge pressure		
PDA	patent ductus arteriosus	VO_2	oxygen consumption
PFO	patent foramen ovale	VSD	ventricular septal defect
PGE	prostaglandin E	WHO	World Health Organization
PH	pulmonary hypertension	WPW	Wolff–Parkinson–White
PICU	paediatric intensive care unit		
PJRT	permanent junctional reciprocating tachycardia		

Cardiac morphology

Sequential segmental analysis

The chambers of the heart and associated vessels are named according to their morphological features rather than by the position within the chest. As an example, the morphological right atrium (RA) has a broad-based atrial appendage whereas the morphological left atrium (LA) has a narrow, finger-like appendage. The usual arrangement of atria, bronchi, lungs, and abdominal organs is shown in Fig. 1.1. 'Mirror-image' arrangement refers to the positions of all of the organs being left–right reversed. However, in some other situations there is over-representation of either right-sided structures (right atrial isomerism) or left-sided structures (left atrial isomerism).

When the heart is being assessed, it is essential to begin with the atrial arrangement, and then to move through the connections of the heart in a stepwise fashion. This is known as *sequential segmental analysis*. Performing this systematically involves knowledge of the characteristic features of each part of the anatomy (Box 1.1).

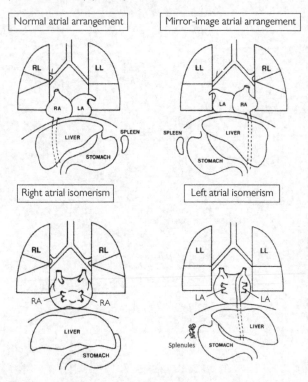

Fig. 1.1 Atrial arrangement, bronchi, abdomen, and isomerism. LL, left lung; RL, right lung.

Box 1.1 Morphological features used to define each cardiac chamber

Right atrium
- Broad-based appendage.
- Pectinate muscles extend into atrial wall.
- Usually receives inferior vena cava (IVC)/superior vena cava (SVC).

Left atrium
- Narrow appendage.
- Pectinate muscles confined to appendage.
- Usually receives pulmonary veins (PVs).

Right ventricle
- Tricuspid valve (trileaflet, septal attachments, more apical insertion).
- Coarse trabeculations.
- Moderator band.

Left ventricle
- Mitral valve (bileaflet, no septal attachments, inserted further from apex).
- Fine trabeculations.
- No moderator band.

Normally, the RA connects to the right ventricle (RV), which connects to the pulmonary artery (PA), and the LA connects to the left ventricle (LV), which connects to the aorta. If a segment connects normally to the next (e.g. RA connects to RV) then this connection is *concordant*. If, however, the RA connects to the LV, this connection is *discordant*. If no connection exists at all then the connection is *absent*. If both atriums connect to the same ventricle, this is known as *double inlet*.

In some settings it may be difficult to ascribe one segment to another. For example, in tetralogy of Fallot the aorta overrides the ventricular septum; in this situation many clinicians apply the '50% rule', i.e. if >50% of the aorta arises from the LV the connection is concordant. In *double-outlet right ventricle* (DORV), both great arteries arise completely or predominantly from the RV, but the precise anatomical arrangement is highly variable. If an arterial valve is *atretic* then, by convention, the artery is not committed to either ventricle. *Transposition of the great arteries* (TGA) means that the aorta arises completely/predominantly from the morphological RV and the PA arises completely/predominantly from the morphological LV, i.e. *discordant ventriculoarterial connections*.

Worked examples of sequential segmental analysis in two types of congenital heart disease (CHD) are shown in Fig. 1.2.

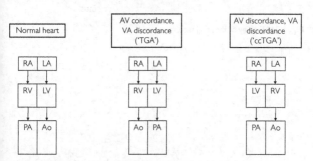

Fig. 1.2 Sequential segmental analysis of normal heart, TGA, and congenitally corrected TGA (ccTGA). Ao, aorta.

Septal structures

Atrial septum

The normal features of the atrial septum can be assessed by visualization *en face* from the RA or LA. The atrial septum is best shown in the anatomical position, i.e. as if an individual is standing up. Hence, the SVC enters the superior aspect of the RA and the IVC the inferior aspect. Inferiorly, the mouth of the coronary sinus can be seen entering the RA. Note that the right PVs pass behind the RA to enter the LA on the other side of the atrial septum. The key landmarks are shown in Fig. 1.3.

Ventricular septum

Landmarks on the ventricular septum and the classification of portions of the ventricular septum are classically viewed from the RV aspect. The ventricular septum can be divided into the small membranous septum and the much larger muscular septum (which itself can be divided into inlet, outlet, and trabecular portions). The key landmarks are shown in Fig. 1.4.

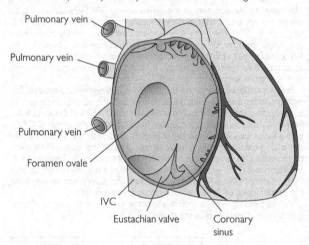

Pulmonary vein

Pulmonary vein

Pulmonary vein

Foramen ovale

IVC

Eustachian valve

Coronary sinus

Fig. 1.3 Anatomy of the atrial septum.

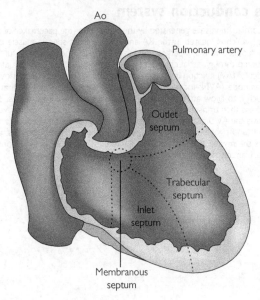

Fig. 1.4 Anatomy of the ventricular septum.

The conduction system

The cardiac impulse is generated by the sinus node (the pacemaker of the heart), which is located in the RA and formed from specific muscle cells richly supplied with sympathetic and vagus nerves. The impulse is further conducted through atrial chambers by atrial musculature. Once the atrio-ventricular (AV) junction is reached, the impulse is delayed by the atrioventricular node (AVN; located in the interatrial septum within the 'triangle of Koch'), to allow atrial chambers to contract and fill the ventricles. The impulse is then transmitted along the interventricular septum to both ventricles via the AV bundle (the bundle of His). The bundle of His divides into the left and right bundle branches, serving the respective ventricles, and enters the myocardium as the Purkinje fibres. This results in synchronous ventricular contraction from the apex towards the base of the heart.

Evaluation of clinical presentations

Heart murmurs

These represent audible blood flow. They should always be interpreted in conjunction with other clinical features.

The presence of a heart murmur does not always signify pathology and significant pathology can be present in the absence of a murmur

Top tips

- The nature of a murmur will be determined by the anatomy and flow conditions that create it.
- Areas of auscultation overlap in neonates and younger children.
- More likely to be pathological when associated with other clinical signs.
- More than one type of murmur can be present simultaneously.

Description of murmurs

- Timing within the cardiac cycle:
  - Systolic (ejection systolic or pansystolic).
  - Diastolic.
  - Continuous.
- Loudness on a scale of 1–6:
  - 1—Quiet.
  - 2—Clearly audible.
  - 3—Loud but not associated with a precordial thrill.
  - 4—Loud with a palpable precordial thrill.
  - 5—Very loud.
  - 6—Audible without a stethoscope.
- Location of maximal intensity on chest wall.
- Areas of radiation.

Anatomy and physiology of murmurs

- Systolic murmur—due to ejection of blood from ventricle in systole:
  - Ventricle ejecting blood back through the inlet valves: *tricuspid or mitral regurgitation*.
  - Ventricle ejecting blood across the outlet valves: *Aortic stenosis (AS) or pulmonary stenosis* (PS).
  - Ventricle ejecting blood across a hole in the ventricular septum: *ventricular septal defect* (VSD).
  - Systolic flow across a narrow blood vessel (e.g. coarctation).
  - Increased blood flow across a normal structure (e.g. pulmonary flow murmur of an atrial septal defect (ASD)).
- Diastolic murmur—noise of blood filling ventricle in diastole:
  - Narrowing or increased blood flow across inlet valves: *tricuspid or mitral stenosis*.
  - Regurgitant flow back into ventricles from incompetent outlet valves: *aortic or pulmonary regurgitation*.

Common types of systolic murmur

Innocent flow murmurs

- Very common, heard in many healthy children, most commonly in infants and toddlers.
- Often heard when there is a raised cardiac output (fever, tachycardia secondary to other systemic illness, anaemia).
- Variable—may change with body position (lying vs sitting) or may be audible at some times and not others.

Features

- Up to 3/6 loudness.
- Systolic—ejection or mid.
- Usually left sternal edge—upper to lower.
- No associated thrill.
- Not diastolic.
- 'Musical' or 'blowing' in character.
- Sometimes a continuous low-pitched venous hum.
- No other associated cardiac signs.

Aortic stenosis (AS) murmur

- Cause: narrowing of the left ventricular outflow tract (LVOT), aortic valve, or ascending aorta.
- Timing: ejection systolic.
- Loudness: often loud and associated with a thrill.
- Location and radiation:
  - Typically right upper sternal edge.
  - May radiate into neck.
  - Subaortic obstruction murmurs heard lower on chest, more to left.
  - Supravalvar aortic murmurs heard higher on chest, more to right.
- Other features:
  - Harsh murmur of blood being ejected across a narrowing.
  - The tighter the narrowing, the higher pitched the murmur.

Aortic arch murmur

- Cause: aortic coarctation.
- Timing: early to mid-systolic murmur as blood passes through coarctation segment. Diastolic continuation of flow means murmur may taper into diastole, especially when heard in the back.
- Loudness: often soft.
- Location: left upper sternal edge and between shoulder blades.

Pulmonary stenosis murmur

- Cause: narrowing of the right ventricular outflow tract (RVOT), pulmonary valve, or pulmonary arterial tree, or relative narrowing caused by increased pulmonary blood flow (e.g. ASD).
- Timing: ejection systolic.
- Location and radiation:
  - Typically upper left sternal edge.
  - May radiate to lung fields.
  - Subpulmonary stenosis murmur louder lower in chest.
  - Can be louder in lung fields if branch narrowing predominates.

- Other features if due to increased pulmonary blood flow (e.g. ASD or partial anomalous pulmonary veins):
  - Softer blowing quality.
  - Fixed splitting of second heart sound due to fixed delay in pulmonary valve closure.
  - Flow murmurs due to volume loading may have RV precordial heave and/or mid-diastolic tricuspid inflow murmur.

Mitral regurgitation murmur
- Timing: pansystolic.
- Location: apical radiating to the left axilla.
- Other features:
  - High pitched due to high-velocity jet.
  - Louder murmur usually indicates more severe regurgitation.
  - LV heave (palpable at apex).
  - Diastolic mitral inflow murmur (due to stenosis or increased blood flow).

Tricuspid regurgitation murmur
- Timing: pansystolic.
- Loudness: usually soft as RV ejects at lower pressure.
- Location: left lower sternal edge, sometimes radiates across to right.
- Other features:
  - Pitch becomes lower as magnitude of regurgitation increases.
  - Tricuspid diastolic inflow murmur if significant volume of regurgitation.
  - Pulsatile liver and distended central veins when severe.

VSD murmur
- Timing: pansystolic (may be short early systolic if very small defect).
- Loudness: inversely proportional to defect size.
- Location: along left sternal edge—depending on the position of the VSD.

Common types of diastolic murmur

Aortic regurgitation murmur
- Timing: diastolic.
- Loudness: usually quieter and higher pitched than aortic systolic murmur.
- Location: heard from aortic valve down into the LV (i.e. along left sternal edge).

Pulmonary regurgitation murmur
- Timing: diastolic.
- Location: from left upper sternal edge radiating down the left sternal edge.
- Often associated with previous interventions (e.g. pulmonary valvotomy or tetralogy repair).

Mitral stenosis murmur
- Timing: diastolic.
- Location: apical to left lower sternal edge.
- May be late systolic accentuation when severe stenosis due to atrial contraction.

Tricuspid stenosis murmur
- Cause: more commonly due to increased flow across a normal tricuspid valve (e.g. large ASD or partial anomalous pulmonary venous drainage) rather than true tricuspid valve stenosis.
- Timing: diastolic.
- Location: right and left lower sternal edge.

Common types of continuous murmur

Patent ductus arteriosus (PDA) murmur
- Timing: continuous.
- Location: left upper sternal edge beneath the clavicle.
- Nature of the murmur depends on the size of the duct, pulmonary artery pressure (PAP), and the magnitude of the shunt.
- Small defects may just have a high-pitched systolic component.
- As the duct becomes larger, the murmur is audible into diastole.
- Moderate to large ducts with high shunt magnitude have loud cyclical continuous murmur ('machinery murmur').
- Very large unrestrictive ducts or those in neonates may have a quieter murmur as there is less turbulence and equivalence of pulmonary and systemic arterial pressures.

Aortopulmonary collateral artery murmur
- Timing: continuous.
- Location: heard posteriorly in the lung fields.
- Almost always associated with complex cyanotic disease with abnormal pulmonary vasculature.

Aortopulmonary shunt (surgical) murmur
- Timing: continuous.
- Location: right or left upper sternal edge depending upon site of shunt.
- Pitch and volume relate to shunt size and PA flow.
- Absence of murmur with severe cyanosis in this setting is a clinical emergency, as this may indicate shunt blockage.

Heart failure

Heart failure in children describes a clinical syndrome where the heart is not able to pump blood to the tissues of the body as effectively as it should. In neonates and infants, it is usually characterized by:

- Breathlessness
- Poor feeding
- Failure to thrive
- Pallor
- Hepatomegaly
- Tachycardia.

Peripheral or dependent oedema is a rare and late sign in neonates and young children. Other clinical signs will depend upon the underlying cause.

Heart failure in children can be considered in three broad and *not* mutually exclusive categories:

1. Excessive pulmonary blood flow.
2. Left heart obstruction.
3. Pump failure.

See Table 2.1 for differential diagnosis of heart failure depending on age at presentation

Table 2.1 Differential diagnoses of heart failure depending on age at presentation

Presenting age	Differential diagnosis
Immediate neonatal period	Critical left heart disease
	Neonatal myocardial infarction
	Neonatal myocarditis
Neonatal to 6 weeks	Left-to-right shunt
	Myocarditis
6 weeks to 3 months	Left-to-right shunt
	ALCAPA
	Myocarditis
	Cardiomyopathy
3 months to 1 year	Cardiomyopathy
	ALCAPA
	Myocarditis
Older than 1 year	Cardiomyopathy
	Acquired heart disease

1. Excessive pulmonary blood flow

Caused by CHD resulting in a *large* left-to-right shunt, usually ventricular or arterial level:

- VSD/atrioventricular septal defect (AVSD).
- PDA.
- Aorto-pulmonary window.
- Unobstructed total anomalous pulmonary venous return.

(Rarely atrial level shunt, unless there is involvement of pulmonary veins.)

The magnitude of pulmonary blood flow is determined by the size of the defect and the pulmonary vascular resistance (PVR). During the early neonatal period PVR is elevated, limiting the shunt. As the PVR falls in the first weeks after delivery, pulmonary blood flow increases, resulting in increasing symptoms with most babies presenting by 6–8 weeks.

As pulmonary blood flow increases, there is:
• Increasing pulmonary vascular congestion
• Increasing respiratory effort
• Breathlessness on exertion (feeding) progressing to breathlessness at rest
• Increased cardiac work and resting tachycardia
• Increased calorie consumption
• Reduced calorie intake due to elevated work of breathing limiting feeding.

Clinical features
• History:
  • Typically well initially but increasingly difficult to feed.
  • Symptoms often attributed to other cause—reflux, milk intolerance, or upper respiratory tract infection.
  • May present with respiratory infection.
• Examination:
  • Tachycardia.
  • Pulses palpable—full with PDA, may be weaker with other shunts.
  • Precordial and subxiphoid heave.
  • Murmur may be quiet or non-specific.
  • Associated respiratory distress.
  • Evidence of poor growth.
• Key investigations:
  • Chest X-ray (CXR): enlarged heart and plethoric lung fields.
  • Electrocardiogram (ECG): tachycardia and biventricular hypertrophy, superior axis in an AVSD.
  • Transthoracic echocardiogram (TTE): identifies underling lesion.

Differential diagnosis
Important overlap in symptoms (especially early and acute presentation) with:
• Sepsis
• Inherited metabolic disease.

Management
Specifics of management will vary depending on local preferences and policies. Broadly, treatment addresses:
• Nutrition:
  • Specialist nutritional support, with high-calorie supplements.
  • Nasogastric feeding.
  • Treatment of associated gastro-oesophageal reflux.
• Cardiac:
  • Diuretics (usually loop and potassium-sparing diuretic together).

- If surgical correction is not imminent, consider systemic vasodilator (angiotensin-converting enzyme inhibitor (ACEi) in ward or outpatient setting, milrinone in high dependency unit (HDU)/ paediatric intensive care unit (PICU)).
- Ultimately, the goal is to correct the underlying abnormality.
- Respiratory:
  - Use respiratory support as clinically required.
  - Nurse in air: oxygen will further lower PVR and increase SVR, increasing the shunt and worsening the patient's clinical condition.
  - Hypoxia is not expected and requires additional investigation for cause.
- Parental support—additional needs of the parents and wider family should be considered:
  - Information on diagnosis and management.
  - Specialist nursing support—in hospital or community.
  - Psychological support.
  - Support for siblings.

Long-term prognosis for the majority of left-to-right shunts causing heart failure is excellent with normal health and lifespan anticipated if there are no residual defects following repair.

Systemic-to-venous shunts

Although large arteriovenous shunts (e.g. vein of Galen, large haemangioma) are similar to the left-to-right shunts detailed above, there are important clinical differences:

- The shunt is not modified by the PVR so symptoms and presentation are usually in the neonatal period.
- The increased volume through the circulation involves both the right and left sides of the heart.
- Diuretics may provide some symptomatic relief, but systemic vasodilation less so.
- Early treatment is required.

2. Left heart obstruction

Congenital obstructive abnormalities of the left side of the heart impact the circulation by:

- Limiting systemic blood flow.
- Increasing LA and pulmonary venous pressure.

More common abnormalities include:

- Aortic valve stenosis
- Coarctation of the aorta.

Less common abnormalities include:

- Supra-mitral membrane
- Cor triatriatum
- Mitral valve stenosis.

Clinical features will depend upon the degree of obstruction with more critical obstructions presenting earlier.

Treatment
- Clinical stabilization where necessary.
- Prostaglandin for critical obstructive lesions.
- Diuresis can be useful as an aid to stabilization.
- Intervention to address the underlying abnormality.

3. Pump failure

Characterized by poor left (or systemic) ventricular function. As with left heart obstruction there is failure to maintain adequate systemic perfusion coupled with elevation of the left ventricular end-diastolic pressure (LVEDP), LA pressure, and pulmonary venous pressure. Causes of pump failure include:
- Acute myocarditis
- Cardiomyopathy
- Neonatal myocardial infarction
- Coronary artery abnormality:
  - Anomalous origin of the left coronary artery from the pulmonary artery (ALCAPA)
  - Other coronary abnormality
- Other lesions resulting in inefficient pump function:
  - Severe mitral regurgitation
  - Severe aortic regurgitation.

Clinical features are variable depending upon the aetiology. Typical presentations include the following:

Myocarditis
(See p. 227.)
- Short history of breathlessness, lethargy, and pallor.
- Older children may complain of chest pain and/or palpitations.
- Usually a prodromal illness (viral or gastroenterological).

Cardiomyopathy
(See p. 224.)
- More insidious presentation over weeks to months.
- Increasing lethargy, tiredness, poor appetite, and irritability.
- In younger children, difficulty with feeding.
- Breathlessness on exertion.
- Orthopnoea and oedema are rare, but more likely if also RV failure.
- Presenting event may be a minor respiratory infection.

ALCAPA
(See p. 36.)
- Often insidious presentation over the first few months of life.
- Lethargy, poor feeding, failure to thrive, and recurrent respiratory symptoms.
- May have episodes of unexplained crying/pain due to angina.
- Usually well at birth and for first weeks of life until PVR decreases.

More information on heart muscle disease can be found in Chapter 11.

Cyanosis

Dusky blue discoloration of the skin or mucus membranes representing deoxygenated haemoglobin (Hb) 3–5 g/dL. Usually corresponds to oxygen saturations of <85%.

Central (e.g. of the tongue)
Causes include:
- Lung disease with inadequate oxygen exchange (often correctable by increasing the inspired oxygen)
- Shunting from pulmonary to systemic circulation (cyanosis is not reversed by increasing the inspired oxygen)
- Inadequate oxygen uptake (e.g. disorders of Hb, high altitude).

Peripheral cyanosis (perioral cyanosis common in children)
- Due to increased oxygen extraction from the capillary bed.
- May have normal transcutaneous saturations.

Causes include:
- Peripheral vasoconstriction
- Low cardiac output
- Venous stasis.

Clinical presentation

Cyanosis can be difficult to detect, especially with darker skin colours, in the presence of jaundice, or in poor light. In infants and children skin takes on a grey/dusky hue.
- More evident in polycythaemia.
- Less evident in anaemia.

Examination should focus on evidence of cardiac or respiratory disease.

Pulse oximetry

Measure of Hb oxygen saturation, expressed as SpO_2. *It is not a measure of arterial PO_2.* Transitive pulse oximeter emits light at two wavelengths:
- Red light at 660 nm.
- Infrared light at 940 nm.

Deoxygenated blood allows more infrared light to pass through and absorb red, whereas oxygenated blood absorbs infrared and allows red light to pass through. The amount of light in each wavelength transmitted to a sensor is measured and the processor converts this to a continuous signal for arterial blood. It is less accurate with:
- Darker skin colours
- Hypoperfusion
- Thickened skin
- Movement
- When saturations are <80%.

Hyperoxia test

Used to determine whether cyanosis in an infant is due to respiratory disease or a right-to-left shunt. This is a measure of change in oxygen content in 100% inspired oxygen.
1. Measurement of arterial PaO_2 in room air.
2. Give 100% oxygen for 10 minutes then repeat arterial PaO_2.
3. Infants with a right-to-left shunt will seldom be able to raise the PaO_2 to >100 mmHg or 13.3 kPa.

Transcutaneous oxygen saturations are not a measure of oxygen content. An increase in arterial saturations to >95% in 100% oxygen is not a negative hyperoxia test and does not exclude CHD.

Neonatal screening for congenital heart disease

Pulse oximetry in the asymptomatic neonate has been proposed as a method for screening for CHD. The baby passes screening where:
- Saturations in right arm are 95% or greater, and
- There is a difference of 3% or less between the arm and the foot.

Repeat screening may be necessary on up to three occasions. Failed screening prompts clinical assessment:
- Clinical indicators of CHD.
- Assessment sepsis or respiratory infection.
- When there are features of CHD or absence of other clinical causes of hypoxia then an echocardiogram is required.

Saturation measurement after 24 hours of age decreases false-positive rate. Preductal (right arm) and postductal saturations (leg) are recommended.

Differential saturations in the newborn

Measurement of pre- and postductal saturations in the newborn provides information on potential CHD or can be used to monitor known CHD. Differential saturations may occur when there is a patent arterial duct with flow from the PA to the aorta, directed to the lower limbs.
- Normal preductal and lower postductal (indicates right-to-left flow at the arterial duct):
  - Persistent pulmonary hypertension of newborn.
  - Aortic obstruction at level of arch (coarctation or interruption).
- Low preductal and higher postductal saturations:
  - Transposition of the great arteries, with PA to aortic flow at the arterial duct (pathognomonic).

Note: in duct-dependent pulmonary circulations where flow is systemic to pulmonary, a saturation differential is not expected.

Cyanosis in the older child

Long-term cyanosis is almost always due to CHD. Although many are oper-
ated, in some a right-to-left shunt may persist:
- Single-ventricle circulation.
- Complex pulmonary atresia.

This is a multisystem disorder with significant morbidity, causing:
- Erythrocytosis and elevated haematocrit secondary to hypoxia
- Thrombocytopenia
- Disordered coagulation with risk of bleed and thrombus
- Risk of neurological complications (cerebral abscess, stroke)
- Renal impairment
- Gout
- Gallstones
- Acne
- Clubbing
- Skeletal abnormalities.

Perioral cyanosis

This is a common paediatric finding. It is a form of acrocyanosis with peripheral vasoconstriction, and increased oxygen extraction as blood takes
longer to pass through blood vessels. May be associated with a history of
cyanosis in extremities. Usually involves skin around mouth and upper lip,
usually not mucus membranes. May be precipitated by:
- Viral upper respiratory tract infection
- Cold environment
- Temperature change
- In many cases there is no obvious trigger.

In the clinically well child with no cardiac signs and normal oxygen saturations, no further investigation is required.

Abnormalities of haemoglobin

Hb comprises four peptide units, two alpha and two beta, with an iron-
containing haem group at its centre. Abnormalities of Hb can impact
oxygen-carrying capacity.
- Methaemoglobinaemia—iron converted from ferrous (2^+) to ferric (3^+)
  state to which oxygen cannot bind:
  - Associated with oxidizing agents (e.g. benzocaine).
  - Congenital methaemoglobinaemia (autosomal recessive mutation in
    the cytochrome b5 reductase enzyme gene).
  - Reversed with methylene blue.
- Sulfhaemoglobinaemia:
  - Irreversible binding of sulphur to haem complex.
  - Drug induced—containing sulphonamides.
  - Ingestion of industrial chemicals.

Palpitations

Palpitations represent the sensation of the heart beating fast or irregularly. Common in children and descriptions will vary according to the child's age and ability to articulate what they are experiencing.

> The sensation of palpitations is often described as 'chest pain'—a careful history is required to distinguish between the two

In the majority, palpitations do not represent cardiac disease and are a consequence of physiological elevation of the heart rate (HR) due to:
• Fever
• Anxiety
• Exercise
• Anaemia.

Importantly, patients with a significant rhythm disturbance may not describe palpitations at all.

Clinical approach

History
A careful history is the most valuable and informative tool when assessing a child with palpitations. Ask the child to:
• Describe in their own words what they are experiencing
• Tap out the rate and rhythm of what they feel.

With respect to the palpitations themselves consider:
• How long have they been occurring for?
• How exactly do they start?
• How long do they last?
• How do they end?
• Has the child found a way to make it stop (e.g. modified Valsalva)?
• How frequently do they occur?
• In what environment do they happen?
• Has the child or family noted a pattern?

Associated symptoms that might indicate a cardiac cause include:
• Chest pains (separate to the sensation of palpitations)
• Dizziness
• Fainting
• Observed colour change.

Other aspects to consider in the history:
• Impact of the palpitations on child:
  • Limitations on activities.
  • Time off school.
• Fluid intake and diet:
  • Is the child remaining adequately hydrated, including at school (fear of going to the toilet means some children will avoid drinking)?

* Are they remaining well hydrated during exercise?
* Ingestion of stimulants—caffeine, high-energy drinks.
* Medication.
* Exercise patterns, how much physical activity does the child do?
* Family history, especially CHD, arrhythmia, pacing, and sudden unexplained death.
* Emotional well-being: careful questioning to gauge well-being in home or school environments.
* Consider other symptoms that may indicate alternate medical causes (e.g. anaemia, hyperthyroidism).

Examination

Clinical examination is most often normal. Check HR, transcutaneous oxygen saturations, and blood pressure (BP). If there are signs of heart disease, then an echocardiogram is indicated. Consider other signs of systemic disease.

Not all children with palpitations require further investigation if there is a clear non-cardiac cause evident in the history.

Investigations

Blood tests

Testing will depend on history and examination findings. Possible cause of palpitations include:
* Anaemia
* Thyroid abnormalities
* Consider vitamin D deficiency in high-risk populations.

12-lead ECG

A resting 12-lead ECG is usually normal. However, it is helpful to demonstrate:
* Normal sinus rhythm
* Absence of pre-excitation (this may be intermittent)
* Hypertrophy
* Repolarization abnormalities.

TTE

To exclude underlying CHD or cardiomyopathy.

Heart rhythm monitoring
See ambulatory ECG section in Chapter 4 p. 100
The purpose of recording is to determine the heart rhythm during symptoms—either to prove the presence of an arrhythmia or to demonstrate that symptoms do not represent an arrhythmia.

The clinical history examination findings and ECG will determine which form of event monitoring would be most informative. Ideally, the child should experience symptoms during the recording.

- *Holter monitoring*: usually 24–72 hours. Occasionally for longer (up to 14 days); however, the stickers can cause skin irritation. This will provide a three-channel ECG recording for the duration of the recording. Useful when:
  - Symptoms are frequent and likely to occur during the period of monitoring
  - Patient is unlikely to be compliant with specific event monitoring.
- *Event monitoring*: also known as external loop recorders, useful in the setting of occasional symptoms, especially in those where the history is more suggestive of a tachyarrhythmia. These devices usually involve the recording of a single-channel ECG through each hand (usually thumb) during symptoms. Recordings can be stored on the machine for analysis by the issuing department on its return.
- *Smartphone-enabled event monitoring*: commercial devices are freely available that provide a single-channel recording—either through a standalone device or incorporated into a phone case. These devices often have analysis undertaken by the commercial provider and then provided to the patient/investigating institution.
- *Smartwatch ECG analysis*: as smartwatch technology improves, case reports are emerging of their use in the detection of rhythm abnormalities in neonates and young children.
- *Implantable loop recorders*: although available these are not used routinely for the investigation of palpitations in children. They are used more frequently for investigation of syncope or as part of a monitoring strategy in complex arrhythmia.

Treatment

The focus of treatment is addressing the underlying cause. This will include an emphasis on:
- Reassurance based on history or investigations.
- Maintaining good diet and hydration.
- Exercise.
- Treatment of underlying medical illness or deficiency.

When palpitations are due to underlying anxiety or emotional stressors, these will need additional help to address. Local resources will vary but children and families may benefit from:
- Counselling available through school or general practitioner
- Community paediatrics
- Clinical psychology
- Child and Adolescent Mental Health Services.

Where an arrhythmia has been documented, this will be treated according to the rhythm diagnosis (see Chapter 10).

Syncope

Syncope in children is common, peaking in the teenage years. The vast majority of cases are benign. Syncope describes the acute loss of consciousness and tone followed by a spontaneous recovery. This may be preceded by symptoms such as:

- Dizziness
- Sweating
- Visual abnormalities (black spots in vision, sensation of tunnel vision)
- Auditory abnormalities (sounds becoming muffled or distant).

In the majority of children syncope reflects either a vasovagal or an orthostatic postural event. The minority of children with syncope have a cardiac cause. A detailed history (including bystander information) will identify cardiac red flags (Box 2.1) and identify those that merit further investigation.

> **Box 2.1 Cardiac red flags for syncope**
> - No prodromal symptoms.
> - Associated with palpitations and chest pain (careful history).
> - Previous cardiac history.
> - Family history of sudden death, arrhythmia, pacing.
> - Syncope when agitated/stressed.
> - Syncope during exercise.*
>
> * Syncope on exercise refers to collapse mid- or on immediate cessation of activity. Syncope once exercise has concluded and the child is recovering is most often a consequence of poor hydration and a vasovagal response.

Causes of syncope

The most common causes of syncope in children are autonomic, such as:
- Vasovagal (also known as neurocardiogenic)
- Orthostatic
- Reflex anoxic syncope (Box 2.2)
- Postural orthostatic tachycardia syndrome (POTS) (Box 2.3).

Cardiac causes include:
- Genetic abnormalities resulting in ventricular arrhythmias:
  - Long QT syndrome (LQTS)
  - Brugada syndrome
  - Catecholaminergic ventricular tachycardia (CPVT)
- Other tachy/brady arrhythmias:
  - Supraventricular tachycardia (SVT)
  - Complete heart block
- Structural heart disease, e.g. AS
- Previously operated structural CHD
- Cardiomyopathies:
  - Dilated cardiomyopathy (DCM)
  - Hypertrophic cardiomyopathy (HCM)
  - Arrhythmogenic right ventricular cardiomyopathy (ARVC)

Box 2.2 Reflex anoxic syncope

Also referred to as reflex anoxic seizures. Describes a sudden loss of consciousness in response to noxious stimulus. Excessive vagal stimulation resulting in transient cardiac standstill. Usually seen in infants and toddlers <5 years of age but can occur at any age.

Characterized by:
- Sudden loss of consciousness
- Extreme pallor, often dark around eyes
- Increased tone with clenched jaw and fine tonic clonic shaking
- As HR recovers, the body relaxes
- Child regains consciousness
- May be very emotional/sleepy for several hours afterwards.

Treatment is focused on supportive management, with careful avoidance of triggers without limiting activities. Education and support for caregivers is vital.

Frequent recurrent episodes can be treated with:
- Anticholinergics (e.g. glycopyrronium, atropine, hyoscine)
- Insertion of permanent pacemaker can be considered when frequent and severe.

Box 2.3 Postural orthostatic tachycardia syndrome

POTS involves chronic symptoms of orthostatic intolerance (over 6 months), including the following experienced while standing:
- Palpitations.
- Presyncope.
- Headaches.
- Fatigue.
- Pallor.

Diagnostic criteria focus on chronic symptoms, together with excessive HR increase on standing (active or tilt testing), above 40 beats per minute (bpm) *without* accompanying hypotension that would define orthostatic hypotension. Treatment options should be tailored to address the multifactorial pathogenesis underlying POTS:
- Increase water and salt intake.
- Avoidance of triggers.
- Increased exercise to avoid physical deconditioning.
- Similar to reflex syncope, medication (e.g. midodrine) should be reserved as second line after initial lifestyle measures have been tried with support from family and medical team. Ivabradine may have a role in those where the tachycardia symptoms predominate.

- Pulmonary hypertension.

  Other non-cardiac causes include:
- Severe anaemia
- Hypoglycaemia
- Seizure disorder

- Migraine
- Narcolepsy
- Drug or toxin induced (e.g. alcohol)
- Pregnancy
- Functional disorder.

Clinical approach to syncope

History

A thorough history is the most important aspect of clinical assessment. Elements of history should include:
- Whether there was loss of consciousness with a fall to the ground
- A detailed account of events leading up to event
- A step-by-step articulation of symptoms to elicit if any prodromal symptoms: 'What did you feel first?', 'Then what happened next?'
- If possible, witness account of event:
  - What did the child do prior to the faint?
  - Physical features
  - Duration of loss of consciousness
  - Nature of recovery
  - Presence or absence of abnormal movements
- Fluid intake and diet—be quite specific about daily fluid volume:
  - E.g. if uses water bottle, what volume is it and how much is ingested over the day
  - When considering diet not just meal frequency but content of meals
- Drug/toxin ingestion
- Family history of syncope and cardiac disease
- Social history including emotional well-being.

Examination

- HR, BP, and saturations at rest.
- Lying and standing HR and BP.
- Signs of undiagnosed structural or acquired heart disease.

Baseline investigations

A 12-lead ECG should be performed on all children who present with syncope. This is to ensure:
- A normal heart rhythm
- Screen for indicators of structural heart disease
- Screen for ventricular hypertrophy
- Identify possible repolarization abnormalities (e.g. long corrected QT interval (QTc)).

Further investigation is not usually required in children with:
- A reassuring history particularly absence of cardiac red flags
- No indicators of other underlying disease
- A normal clinical examination
- A normal 12-lead ECG.

If the history is suggestive of a seizure rather than syncope, then appropriate onward referral is indicated.

Further investigations

Where the history is suspicious of a cardiac cause, or despite a careful history the nature of the syncope is difficult to elucidate, further investigations are indicated:

- TTE: to exclude structural heart disease, cardiomyopathy, or pulmonary hypertension.
- *Holter monitoring*: 24–72-hour recordings are usually unhelpful, unless there are frequent associated palpitations or consideration of POTS.
- Event recording: handheld event recorders are unhelpful—they are unusable in the unconscious patient and a recording after the event is of no diagnostic value.
- Tilt testing: can be useful for selected patients where diagnosis is unclear. The aim is to reproduce the symptoms with demonstration of the associated changes to HR, BP, and vascular tone. Tilt testing can also be helpful in assessment for POTS.
- Implantable loop recorder: insertion of an implantable loop recorder (e.g. Reveal) with download facilities to the cardiac centre can be helpful where there is a high likelihood of a cardiac event (e.g. strong family history or previous cardiac disease).

Treatment of syncope

Most children presenting with syncope can be reassured with no specific treatment or mitigation of obvious triggers. In this case advice should be given regarding:
- Ensuring good hydration
- Maintaining a regular and balanced diet.

An example of avoiding or mitigating triggers is for syncope associated with injections/blood tests—undertake these with the child lying flat, rather than sitting.

Treatment of recurrent vasovagal or orthostatic syncope

Most common in adolescents. The overall strategy is to maintain euvolaemia with adequate fluid and salt intake, and vascular tone with regular exercise. Becoming physically deconditioned tends to exacerbate symptoms.
- Maintain consistent fluid intake throughout the day:
  - 2.5–3 L per day.
  - Avoid stimulants/diuretics (caffeine, high-sugar drinks).
- Optimize salt intake:
  - 5–6 g salt per day (2.5–3 g sodium per day)
- Maintain good vascular tone:
  - Regular aerobic exercise.
  - Isometric exercise to improve muscle tone.
  - Leg exercises (contraction/relaxation of calves and thighs) before standing.

Other measures include:
- Compression stockings
- Elevating head of the bed.

Medical treatment

If conventional approaches fail then medical treatment can be utilized *in addition to the more conservative measures above.*

Fludrocortisone:
- Potent mineralocorticoid.
- Results in fluid retention and elevation in BP.
- Electrolytes need to be monitored.
- Suitable for prescription in primary care.

Midodrine:
- Sympathomimetic agent acting on alpha adrenergic receptors to increase vascular tone.
- Unlicensed in UK for use in children <18 years of age.
- Can be helpful in adolescents—hospital-only prescription.

Beta-blockers (rarely used in children for syncope):
- Propranolol.
- Atenolol.

Chest pain

Chest pain

Chest pain is a common presenting feature *but rarely associated with cardiac disease in children*. It is a common reason for referral to paediatric cardiology outpatient clinics. There is a broad differential diagnosis.

Non-cardiac causes of chest pain

- Idiopathic:
  - Prolonged history.
  - Often psychosocial element.
- Costochondritis:
  - Sharp anterior chest wall pain.
  - Localized tenderness.
- Musculoskeletal:
  - Sometimes reproduced with movement.
  - History muscle injury.
  - Often in adolescence, boys > girls.
  - Precordial catch.
  - Symptoms can be exacerbated by associated vitamin D deficiency.
- Psychological or functional symptoms:
  - Often associated with other non-specific symptoms.
  - Careful history.
  - Exclusion of pathology important to build reassurance.
- Respiratory:
  - Asthma.
  - Pneumonia.
  - Pleural effusion (infective, malignancy).
  - Pneumothorax—if spontaneous, consider Marfan syndrome.
- Gastrointestinal:
  - Gastro-oesophageal reflux.
  - Oesophagitis/gastritis.
  - Gallbladder disease.
- Other causes:
  - Shingles.
  - Breast masses.
  - Skeletal tumours.

Cardiac causes of chest pain

- Carditis—myocarditis, pericarditis, pancarditis, and endocarditis.
- Arrhythmia—SVT or ventricular tachycardia (VT).
- Coronary artery disease:
  - Kawasaki disease (KD).
  - Congenital coronary artery abnormality.
  - Previous CHD surgery involving coronary arteries (e.g. TGA post switch).
- Inherited cardiac disease (e.g. HCM).
- CHD (e.g. late presentation of AS or aortic coarctation).
- Aortic disease (e.g. connective tissue disorders with associated dissection).
- Drug-induced ischaemia (most commonly cocaine).

- Pulmonary embolus (rare in children, usually with prothrombotic risk factors).
- Mitral valve prolapse.
- Pathological causes of chest pain will have a combination of:
  - Additional clinical signs, e.g. murmur of AS or absent femoral pulses in aortic coarctation
  - ECG abnormalities: ischaemia, hypertrophy, pericarditic changes.

Structured approach to evaluation of chest pain

History

- PMH—history of CHD or KD.
- Family history of cardiac disease, aortic abnormalities, or sudden death.
- Medication/drug ingestion.
- Characterization of chest pain:
  Site of pain (left/right, upper/lower).
  Onset (slow/sudden).
  Character (sharp/stabbing/ache).
  Radiation (nil/neck/arm/abdomen).
  Associated (nausea/palpitations/dizzy).
  Timing (rest/exercise/food).
  Exacerbating/relieving (with breathing/analgesia).
  Score (X/10).
- Psychosocial history can be important.

Examination

- Vital signs.
- Chest wall—asymmetry, localized or generalized tenderness.
- Cardiac examination—pulses, heaves, thrills, heart sounds, murmurs.
- Respiratory examination—features of pneumothorax, infection.
- Abdominal examination—masses, distension, epigastric tenderness.

Investigations

- 12-lead ECG—arrhythmia, ischaemia, hypertrophy.
- CXR if clear respiratory signs.
- Vitamin D level in chronic and recurrent pain with risk factors.
- Cardiac enzymes if features of ischaemia.
- Echocardiogram in selected cases.

Treatment of chest pain

- This should be directed towards the underlying cause.
- In most cases reassurance and/or simple analgesic is all that is required.
- Treat vitamin D deficiency.

Structural congenital heart disease

Prevalence of structural congenital heart disease

CHD is the most common group of congenital anomalies. The frequency of individual CHD lesions will vary by geographical region, recording method, and lesion definition. Table 3.1 shows the total birth prevalence for some selected structural CHD lesions recorded by the English National Congenital Anomaly and Rare Disease Registration Service (NCARDRS) in 2019.

Table 3.1 The 2019 birth prevalence of specific CHD lesions

Lesion	Total birth prevalence per 10,000 births	
	Including genetic cases	*Excluding genetic cases*
Aortic valve stenosis/atresia	1.2	1.1
ASD	10.5	8.3
AVSD	5.9	2.4
Coarctation of the aorta	4.8	4.0
DORV	2.0	1.7
Ebstein's anomaly	0.4	0.4
Hypoplastic left heart	3.0	2.7
Interrupted aortic arch	0.4	0.3
Mitral valve abnormalities	1.6	1.3
Patent arterial duct (in term infants only, as only lesion)	0.3	0.3
Pulmonary atresia	1.7	1.4
Pulmonary valve stenosis	3.4	3.2
Tetralogy of Fallot	4.7	3.6
Total anomalous pulmonary venous drainage	1.1	1.0
Transposition of the great arteries	3.2	3.0
Tricuspid atresia	0.9	0.9
VSD	26.1	21.4

Anomalous left coronary artery from the pulmonary artery (ALCAPA)

Anatomy

(See Fig. 3.1.)
- Normally the left coronary artery arises from the left coronary sinus, above the aortic valve.
- ALCAPA is when the left coronary artery arises from the PA.

Physiology

- The ventricular myocardium experiences a 'double hit' of reduced oxygenation (deoxygenated blood from the PA) and impaired perfusion (due to lower perfusion pressure).
- In normal anatomy, blood flow in the coronary arteries is driven by perfusion pressure (the difference between diastolic pressure in aorta and RA pressure).
- As PVR falls, the pressure in the pulmonary trunk falls and in the setting of ALCAPA there is reduced perfusion pressure to the coronary arteries.
- The combination of reduced oxygenation and reduced perfusion leads to impaired contractility.
- To maintain stroke volume the LV dilates which may lead to mitral regurgitation.
- As LVEDP increases above the PA pressure, this leads to reversed flow in the anomalous left coronary artery.
- Collateralization from the right coronary artery may occur.

Clinical features

- Usually presents in early infancy with symptoms/signs of heart failure (see p. 12).

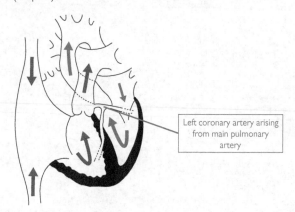

Left coronary artery arising from main pulmonary artery

Fig. 3.1 ALCAPA.

- Pansystolic murmur at lower left sternal edge (variable) if mitral regurgitation present from annular dilatation.
- Arrhythmias may occur.
- If good collateralization, then may present in later childhood with angina/arrhythmias during exercise.

Treatment

- Medical treatment of heart failure with diuretics, and feeding/ respiratory support.
- Timely surgical repair is crucial, with reimplantation of the left coronary artery into the aorta.
- May require postoperative support with extracorporeal membrane oxygenation (ECMO) as a bridge to recovery.
- If mitral valve regurgitation remains, may need mitral valve repair.

Outcome

- Very good postoperative survival.
- May be residual impairment of LV contractility requiring medical management.
- Recovery of LV function may take months or years.

Aortic stenosis (AS)

Anatomy

(See Fig. 3.2.)
- The normal aortic valve consists of an aortic root within which are three leaflets separated by three commissures representing the lines of apposition of the leaflets.
- Narrowing of the valve annulus or the subvalvar/supravalvar regions can occur.
- *Valvar stenosis* (60–75% of AS cases) may be due to:
  - Fusion of the commissures preventing the valve from opening, *or*
  - Dysplastic thickening of the leaflets with reduced mobility, *or*
  - A small annulus.
- Bicuspid aortic valve (present in 2% of the general population) usually represents partial fusion of the leaflets—a true bicuspid valve is rarer. Stenosis is variable and may progress over time.
- *Subvalvar stenosis* (8–30% of AS cases) can be due to a ridge or membrane in the LVOT or from malalignment of the ventricular septum.
- *Supravalvar stenosis* (1–2% of AS cases) is categorized as hourglass, membranous, or tubular in nature.

Associations

- Supravalvar AS is commonly associated with elastin gene mutations such as Williams syndrome (see p. 178).

Physiology

- Obstruction to egress of blood from the LV leading to a pressure-overloaded ventricle, leading to LV hypertrophy and fibrosis.

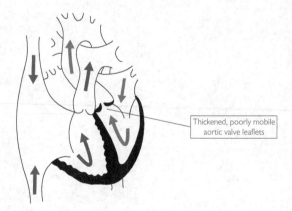

Thickened, poorly mobile aortic valve leaflets

Fig. 3.2 AS.

- Severe stenosis presents soon after birth leading to reduced systemic perfusion, resulting in acidosis and shock.
- Coronary blood flow can be affected in those with supravalvar AS.

Clinical features

- Related to the degree of obstruction.
- Mild AS presents with a soft ejection systolic murmur at the upper right sternal edge radiating to the carotids; there may be a thrill in the suprasternal notch.
- Moderate or severe AS presents with louder harsh murmur ± thrill and leads to LVH and a hyperdynamic precordium.
- Exercise intolerance, chest pain, or syncope are rare presentations.
- In critical AS, presentation is in the newborn, with insufficient cardiac output leading to reduced pulses and perfusion, shock, lactic acidosis, and later to death.

Treatment

- Mild valvar AS can be monitored conservatively.
- Critical AS requires an infusion of prostaglandin E to maintain ductal patency prior to intervention.
- Valvar AS can be treated with either a balloon aortic valvuloplasty or surgical valvotomy. Outcomes are similar.
- Extremely diseased valves may require a surgical valve replacement:
  - A Ross procedure may be performed (see p. 135).
  - Prosthetic aortic valve replacements can also be used but may need anticoagulation.
- Subvalvar or supravalvar AS requires surgery to enlarge the narrowed region.

Outcomes

- AS is a progressive lesion if untreated, with an increased risk of sudden death if severe.
- Following intervention, there is 85% survival at 25 years.
- Aortic root and ascending aortic dilation may require monitoring in longer term.

Aortopulmonary window

Anatomy

(See Fig. 3.3.)
- Communication between ascending aorta and PA trunk.
- Usually no arterial duct.

Associations

- Usually seen in isolation, but 25–50% associated with other lesions (coarctation of aorta, arch interruption, tetralogy of Fallot, TGA, pulmonary atresia, VSD).
- Can be associated with chromosome 22q11 microdeletion (see p. 40).

Physiology

- Unrestrictive communication at arterial level.
- Physiologically similar to large arterial duct.
- When PVR falls, will develop increasing left-to-right shunt, pulmonary over-circulation, and diastolic steal from systemic circulation.

Clinical features

- Large communication often means no murmur in the neonatal period.
- Clinical features of increased pulmonary flow (Qp) develop in the first few weeks of life, as PVR falls.
- Wide pulse pressure.
- If PVR does not fall, may remain asymptomatic or present later with cyanosis.

Treatment

- Medical treatment of high Qp with diuretics and feeding/respiratory support.

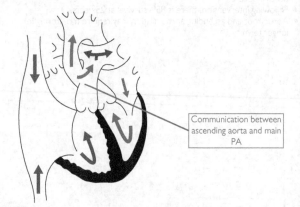

Communication between ascending aorta and main PA

Fig. 3.3 Aortopulmonary window.

- Most cases will require full surgical repair.
- In selected cases device occlusion can be considered.

Outcomes

- Short- and long-term postsurgical survival is excellent.
- A small number of cases require late intervention for acquired right PA stenosis.

Atrial septal defect (ASD)

Anatomy

(See Fig. 3.4.)
- All defects that lead to shunting at the level of the atria are referred to as ASDs.
- *Patent foramen ovale* (PFO): usually considered separately from ASDs, and present in 25–30% of the general population; this is a flap-like communication between the primum and secundum septums.
- Major types of ASDs:
  - *Secundum ASD*: 70% of ASD cases, a defect in the central portion of the atrial septum, in the region of the oval fossa.
  - *Atrioventricular septal defect* (AVSD): atrial component (ostium primum ASD) typically crescent-shaped adjacent to AV valves (see p. 44).
  - *Superior sinus venosus ASD*: superiorly located at the junction of SVC and RA. Right-sided partial anomalous pulmonary venous drainage typically coexists. Inferior sinus venosus ASD very rare.
  - *Coronary sinus defect*: <1% of ASD cases involve unroofing of a portion of the coronary sinus, allowing a communication with the LA.

Physiology

- The flow across an ASD is determined by the compliance and longitudinal function of the RV as well as the size of the defect.
- Usually, a significant pressure gradient does not exist between the two atria and the flow is left to right.
- This causes a degree of pulmonary over-circulation.

Clinical features

- Clinical features depend on the size, position, and number of defects and their cumulative left-to-right shunt.
- Infants will usually be asymptomatic.

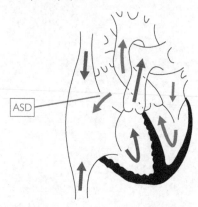

ASD

Fig. 3.4 ASD.

- Frequent chest infections can occur as a result of mildly raised Qp.
- Exercise tolerance reduced in older children.
- Poor feeding and failure to thrive seen in a minority.
- Normal oxygen saturations.
- A hyperdynamic RV impulse may be felt.
- Fixed splitting of the second heart sound, or 'flow' murmur (soft ejection systolic murmur at upper left sternal edge) from relative pulmonary valve stenosis may be auscultated.

Treatment

- Small defects may be managed conservatively.
- Quantifying the ratio of pulmonary to systemic blood flow (Qp:Qs) can be useful to determine the shunt; >2:1 is typically regarded as a significant shunt.
- Diuretics can reduce the volume load on the right heart.
- Surgical closure carries a low risk of mortality but usually requires median sternotomy and bypass.
- Interventional device closure is frequently used for secundum defects depending on size and adjacent rims. There is a small risk of device embolus or early thrombosis. Selected sinus venosus ASDs may be suitable for interventional closure.

Outcomes

- There are excellent outcomes for those repaired in childhood with a mortality rate near zero and a life expectancy near to that of the general population.
- Those with untreated defects carry a risk in later life of pulmonary hypertension, paradoxical embolus, atrial fibrillation (AF), and heart failure.

Atrioventricular septal defect (AVSD)

Anatomy

(See Fig. 3.5.)
- AVSDs (also termed AV canal defects) are defined as a common AV valve guarding a common AV junction. The size of the atrial and ventricular components varies.
- The size of the ventricles may be equal (balanced) or unequal (unbalanced).
- Characterized by superior and inferior bridging leaflets of the AV valve passing across the ventricular septum, fundamentally altering the appearance from normal.

Associations

- Commonest genetic association is trisomy 21 (see p. 175), and a frequent association with laterality disturbance (isomerism).
- Abnormalities of the outflow tracts may coexist, most commonly tetralogy of Fallot.

Physiology

- Depending on the size of ventricular and atrial components of the defect, there is left-to-right shunting of blood.
- As the PVR falls after birth, left-to-right shunting will increase.
- In a minority of cases, there is severe AV valve regurgitation.

Clinical features

- Clinical features are those of heart failure secondary to high pulmonary blood flow (see p. 12).
- In cases with an absent or restrictive ventricular component, presentation may be later due to exercise intolerance, or with an incidental murmur (similar to ASD).

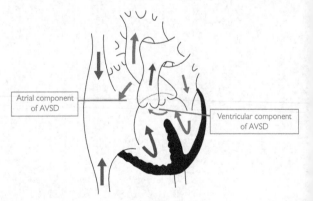

Atrial component of AVSD

Ventricular component of AVSD

Fig. 3.5 AVSD.

Treatment

- Medical treatment of high Qp with diuretics and feeding/respiratory support.
- If there is an unrestrictive ventricular component, surgery is typically undertaken at 3–6 months of age.
- If there is no/restrictive ventricular component, surgery may be deferred until the child is older.
- If there is severe AV valve regurgitation, early surgery (<3 months) may be indicated.

Outcome

- Following complete surgical repair, the cardiac outcome is generally favourable.
- 10–15% of patients may require further surgery on the AV valves following initial repair.

Coarctation of the aorta

Anatomy

(See Fig. 3.6.)
- Narrowing of the aorta, most commonly involving a discrete periductal narrowing.
- Associated hypoplasia of the transverse arch is common (may also have smaller ascending aorta).

Associations

- Can be found in isolation, or associated with other defects (e.g. VSD or TGA).
- 70–75% have a bicuspid aortic valve.
- 'Shone complex' describes multiple left heart stenoses: mitral stenosis (including supramitral membrane), AS (including sub-AS), and coarctation.
- Association with Turner syndrome (see p. 176).

Physiology

- While the PDA is open, there is flow from the aorta to the head and neck vessels and flow from the arterial duct to the lower body (right to left).
- As the PDA closes, there will continue to be flow to the head and neck vessels proximal to the narrowing, but reduced flow distal to the narrowing. The degree of narrowing will dictate the mode of presentation.
- Critical coarctation/arch hypoplasia is duct dependent (see p. 312).

Clinical features

- Most patients present in the neonatal period or in infancy after the arterial duct closes.
- While the duct is open, lower limb saturations < right arm saturations as there may be right-to-left flow from the duct, but the BPs and femoral pulses will remain similar.
- As the duct closes:
  • The saturations will become similar as the right-to-left flow is lost
  • Reduced BP in the lower limbs with reduced femoral pulses

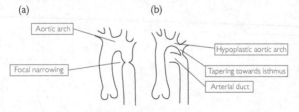

(a)   (b)

Aortic arch

Focal narrowing

Hypoplastic aortic arch

Tapering towards isthmus

Arterial duct

Fig. 3.6 Coarctation of the aorta. (a) Discrete coarctation. (b) Hypoplastic arch with patent arterial duct.

- Reduced gut, liver, and kidney perfusion leading to end-organ dysfunction and shock with breathlessness from pulmonary congestion.
- May have a murmur, often best heard over the left scapula.
- In some cases, may present later with an incidental finding of upper limb BP >20 mmHg higher than lower limb BP and reduced or absent femoral pulses.

Treatment

- Prostaglandin infusion to maintain the arterial duct if necessary.
- In neonates, surgical repair is either via lateral thoracotomy (in isolated coarctation) or median sternotomy (if there is associated arch hypoplasia requiring reconstruction).
- In some infants and older children, catheter intervention with ballooning ± stenting is possible as an alternative to surgery.

Outcomes

- Dependent also on associated conditions.
- Monitoring of arch growth as the child grows is required—many patients will not need a further procedure.
- If there is ongoing narrowing, or the arch fails to grow satisfactorily, then repeat intervention may be required to prevent hypertension: catheter versus surgery depending on anatomy.
- Hypertension in the longer term is an issue, there is a higher risk in those diagnosed later—thought to be an intrinsic issue with aortic vasculature.

Common arterial trunk (truncus arteriosus)

Anatomy

(See Fig. 3.7.)

- A single arterial trunk arises from the ventricles, giving rise to systemic, pulmonary, and coronary circulations.
- This common trunk arises astride a large VSD.
- The truncal valve most commonly has three leaflets but can also have two or four.
- The valve is often dysplastic and can be incompetent or stenotic.
- Classified according to the origin of the PAs (Fig 3.7).
- Usually no arterial duct.

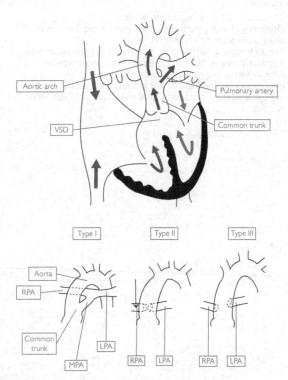

Fig. 3.7 Truncus subtypes. LPA, left pulmonary artery; MPA, main pulmonary artery; RPA, right pulmonary artery.

Associations

- Aortic arch is right sided in around 30%.
- Can be associated with interrupted aortic arch.
- 30% associated with 22q11 microdeletion (see p. 177).

Physiology

- There is a common mixing of oxygenated and deoxygenated blood.
- As PVR falls, there will be increasing Qp.
- Because of the low resistance in the pulmonary circulation, there is diastolic steal from the systemic circulation.

Clinical features

- Usually presents in the first weeks of life with cyanosis, and evidence of pulmonary over-circulation.
- Wide pulse pressure with bounding pulses.
- Murmur (can be variable).

Treatment

- Medical treatment of high Qp, with diuretics and feeding/respiratory support.
- In cases of prematurity or low weight, can consider PA banding in selected cases.
- Aim in most cases is for primary full surgical repair:
  - PAs disconnected from common trunk.
  - Resulting defect in aorta closed with patch.
  - VSD closed with patch to baffle LV to aorta.
  - Continuity between RV and PAs restored, with, e.g. homograft conduit or pericardial patch.

Outcomes

- 92% 30-day and 82% 1-year postoperative survival in the UK.
- Worse survival if associated lesions (e.g. interrupted aortic arch).
- After surgery reintervention to the RV–PA conduit almost inevitable (either transcatheter or surgical replacement), but timing is variable.

Discordant atrioventricular and ventriculoarterial connections (congenitally corrected transposition of the great arteries (ccTGA))

Anatomy

(See Fig. 3.8.)

- There is 'double discordance' of the main cardiac connections, meaning that the RA is connected to the morphological LV and then PA, and the LA is connected to the morphological RV and then aorta.
- The arrangement of the atriums can be usual, or in some cases mirror image.

Associations

- Can exist as an isolated lesion, or in combination with many other CHD lesions including VSDs or abnormalities of an AV or arterial valve (particularly pulmonary stenosis (PS) and Ebstein's anomaly).

Physiology

- In the isolated form, oxygenated blood still enters the aorta (passing through the morphological RV) and deoxygenated blood enters the PA (passing through the morphological LV).
- This means the RV is acting as the systemic ventricle and may start to fail over time.
- Other associated lesions may alter the physiology drastically.

Clinical features

- In isolated cases there may be few or no clinical features, and oxygen saturation will be normal.

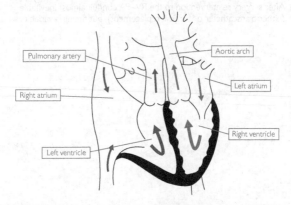

Fig. 3.8 Discordant atrioventricular and ventriculoarterial connections (ccTGA).

- Clinical features are often those of the associated lesions, such as a murmur of a VSD.
- Congenital complete heart block is found in some cases.

Treatment

- This is controversial.
- Some centres undertake a 'double-switch operation' (also known as 'anatomical repair') for isolated cases, i.e. performing both an atrial and arterial switch, making the LV the systemic ventricle. This is not a universal practice, as some feel the benefits do not outweigh the risks.
- Some advocate for PA banding prior to double switch to 'retrain' the LV before switching.
- A 'physiological repair' can be performed for associated lesions, e.g. closing a VSD, but leaving the ventricles with their discordant connections.
- In some, a single-ventricle circulation is the only surgical option.
- In many isolated cases, conservative management is pursued.

Outcomes

- This is highly variable, and in part dependent on associated lesions.
- There are well-described case reports of this lesion being incidentally discovered on autopsy in old age, demonstrating that, for some, conservative management is appropriate.
- Ebstein's anomaly is tolerated poorly, as the tricuspid valve is the systemic AV valve, and associated with high early mortality.

Double-outlet right ventricle (DORV)

Anatomy

(See Fig. 3.9.)
• Both great vessels arise from the RV with a VSD.

Associations

• May be associated with other complex lesions (AVSDs, coarctation of the aorta, abnormal AV valves).

Physiology

• The position of the VSD and arrangement of great vessels dictate the physiology along with degree of obstruction to the outflows.
• Subaortic VSD ('tetralogy of Fallot type', Fig. 3.9a):

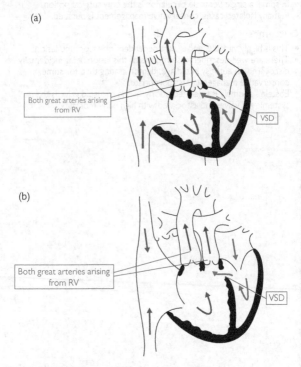

(a)

Both great arteries arising
from RV

VSD

(b)

Both great arteries arising
from RV

VSD

Fig. 3.9 DORV. (a) Tetralogy of Fallot type. (b) Transposition type.

- Blood from the LV streams mostly towards the aorta.
  - Presentation depends on degree of PS, with severe pulmonary obstruction presenting with desaturation (like tetralogy of Fallot) and little or no pulmonary obstruction presenting like a VSD.
- Subpulmonary VSD ('transposition type', Fig. 3.9b):
  - Blood from the LV streams mostly towards the PA.
  - Presents like TGA with lower preductal saturations.
  - Saturations dependent on degree of mixing at atrial, ventricular, and ductal level (see p. 312).
- Doubly committed VSD:
  - Blood can stream to either outflow.
  - Presentation will depend on the degree of obstruction to either outflow.
- Non-committed (remote) VSD:
  - Blood from the LV enters the RV and then both outflows.
  - The VSD is not in close proximity to either outflow tract.
  - Presentation will depend on the degree of obstruction to either outflow.

Clinical features

- Presentation will depend on the position of the VSD and degree of outflow obstruction (see earlier 'Physiology' section).
- Murmur may be present depending on the size of the VSD and outflow obstruction.

Treatment

- Depends on exact anatomical substrate, with some patients needing an initial palliation prior to complete repair:
  - *Severe pulmonary obstruction*: augmentation of pulmonary blood flow (pulmonary valve balloon, arterial shunt, stenting of arterial duct).
  - *Coarctation of the aorta*: surgical repair of coarctation.
  - *Unrestricted pulmonary blood flow*: PA band.
- VSD with pulmonary obstruction may be 'balanced', and not need immediate treatment.
- Full surgical repair is the eventual aim and varies depending on the VSD anatomy.
- Either a biventricular (preferred) or univentricular strategy will be used, depending on the underlying anatomy.

Outcomes

- For biventricular repair, problems seen postoperatively include:
  - Residual right ventricular outflow tract obstruction (RVOTO)
  - Left ventricular outflow tract obstruction (LVOTO) from the position and angle of the LV-to-aorta tunnel
  - Need to replace an RV-to-PA conduit
  - Coronary artery insufficiency from issues during transfer or compression/distortion due to new position
  - Branch PA stenosis if an arterial switch has needed has been performed.

Ebstein's anomaly

Anatomy

(See Fig. 3.10.)
- The normal tricuspid valve is comprised of three leaflets: the anterosuperior, septal, and inferior leaflets.
- Ebstein's anomaly is characterized by apical displacement of the septal and inferior leaflets, coupled with anterosuperior rotation of the plane of the tricuspid valve.
- This leads to 'atrialization' of part of the RV.
- There is a variable degree of tricuspid valve regurgitation, due to deficiency of the septal and/or inferior leaflets with failure of coaptation.
- The anterosuperior leaflet is enlarged, sail-like, and normally inserted.
- Tricuspid valve attachments may extend into the subpulmonary area, causing physical obstruction, and multiple small chordal attachments are characteristic.
- The RV myocardium is typically abnormal causing diastolic dysfunction. There is usually an ASD with variable shunt. Accessory conduction pathways may coexist.

Physiology

- There is tricuspid regurgitation, and this coupled with the reduced function of the RV leads to a reduction in forward flow through the pulmonary valve (sometimes leading to functional pulmonary atresia).
- There is usually right-to-left shunt at atrial level, causing cyanosis.

Clinical features

- There is a wide spectrum of severity which impacts clinical features.
- Cardiomegaly is frequent due to tricuspid valve regurgitation.
- In the neonatal period, cyanosis is the most common presenting feature.

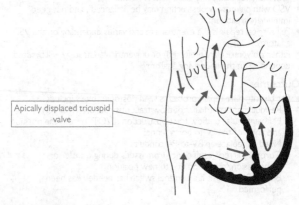

Apically displaced tricuspid valve

Fig. 3.10 Ebstein's anomaly.

- May present as older child or adult with shortness of breath on exercise, cyanosis, or related to arrhythmias (due to accessory pathways).

Treatment

- In the neonatal period, medical support with ventilation, pulmonary vasodilators (e.g. inhaled nitric oxide, sildenafil, supplemental oxygen) are used to lower PVR and encourage forward flow through the right heart.
- Prostaglandin E (PGE) is generally avoided to allow the arterial duct to close and PA pressures to fall, encouraging antegrade flow into pulmonary circulation.
- Once PVR falls, many neonates will have sufficient pulmonary blood flow to defer tricuspid valve surgery until later in life.
- Neonatal tricuspid valve repair is generally not favoured. Blalock–Thomas–Taussig (BTT) shunt insertion to maintain pulmonary blood flow is performed in selected cases.
- Oversewing of the tricuspid valve can be undertaken in severe cases (Starnes procedure), resulting in a univentricular circulation.
- The surgical repair of the tricuspid valve is usually undertaken at >2–3 years of life.
- 'Cone' repair of the tricuspid valve is increasingly favoured to reduce tricuspid regurgitation.
- A Glenn shunt (SVC to branch PA) is used to augment pulmonary blood flow and increase saturations in selected cases.

Outcomes

- Neonates presenting with severe cyanosis and cardiac enlargement ('wall-to-wall heart') have a high mortality rate.
- Those presenting after the neonatal period have a better prognosis.

Hypoplastic left heart syndrome (HLHS)

Anatomy

(See Fig. 3.11.)
- Hypoplasia, stenosis, or atresia of the left heart structures.
- Three main subgroups of 'classical' HLHS:
  - *Mitral and aortic atresia* with slit-like LV.
  - *Mitral stenosis and aortic atresia* with a hypoplastic globular LV. This subgroup is associated with fistulae from the coronary arteries to the ventricular cavity.
  - *Mitral stenosis and aortic stenosis* with a degree of LV hypoplasia.
- Other variants with critical left heart obstruction include DORV with mitral stenosis/atresia, aortic atresia with a VSD, unbalanced AVSD, and critical AS. These variants may have very different management and outcomes to classical HLHS.

Associations

- Associated with genetic conditions in 5–12%.
- Can be seen in Turner syndrome (carrying a poorer prognosis) (see p. 176).
- May be family history of other left heart conditions (e.g. bicuspid aortic valve, coarctation of the aorta).

Physiology

- Pulmonary venous blood passes through the atrial communication to mix with the systemic venous return in the RA to enter the RV and PA.
- Blood flows to the lungs, and to the systemic circulation via the arterial duct (including coronary flow).
- As PVR falls, ductal flow to the lungs increases causing steal from the systemic and coronary circulations, leading to ischaemia and shock.

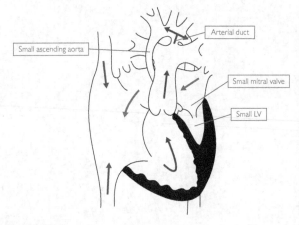

Fig. 3.11 HLHS.

- If the atrial communication is restrictive, there will be obstructed pulmonary venous return causing pulmonary congestion, desaturation, and respiratory distress.
- If the arterial duct starts to close, there will be increased pulmonary blood flow causing pulmonary congestion, breathlessness, and hepatomegaly as well as reduced systemic and coronary flow causing ischaemia and shock.

Clinical features

- If antenatal diagnosis, infants often remain stable if patent atrial communication and arterial duct (on prostaglandin infusion) until the PVR starts to fall around day 2–3, with increasing pulmonary blood flow (and therefore systemic and coronary hypoperfusion).
- Postnatal presentation is usually with ductal closure causing haemodynamic collapse with breathlessness, hepatomegaly, and reduced perfusion, pulses, and BP in all limbs with evidence of end-organ damage (hepatic and renal dysfunction, necrotizing enterocolitis, seizures).
- A murmur may not be present if the duct is unrestrictive and there is no significant tricuspid regurgitation or AS.

Treatment

- Prostaglandin infusion to maintain the patency of the arterial duct.
- In the face of critical atrial communication obstruction, an emergency septal intervention may be required (septostomy, septectomy, septal stent).
- Balancing of the circulations with systemic vasodilators such as milrinone may be required if high Qp.
- Comfort care: this condition cannot be cured, and all procedures are palliative with significant short-, medium-, and long-term morbidity. Non-intervention is therefore a treatment option with involvement of the palliative care team to help with symptoms.
- If active management is pursued, the Norwood procedure is usually the first surgical intervention (see p. 142).
- Hybrid procedure: if the baby is premature and/or low birth weight or in poor condition, then the hybrid procedure is a possible non-bypass initial palliation. Bilateral PA bands with maintenance of prostaglandin or a stent in the arterial duct ± atrial septostomy.
- Primary transplantation: although an option in the US, not a viable option in the UK due to lack of availability of organs.
- Norwood and hybrid procedures are the first steps of palliation towards the Fontan circulation.

Outcomes

- Untreated, HLHS is universally fatal.
- Up to 90% 30-day UK survival following Norwood, but 5–20% interstage mortality after Norwood prior to superior cavopulmonary connection.
- Medium- and longer-term outcomes affected by complications from the Fontan circulation. Most children reach adulthood, but with comorbidities (see Chapter 6).
- At least 1/3 of children with HLHS will have special educational needs or neurodevelopmental issues.

Interrupted aortic arch

Anatomy

(See Fig. 3.12.)
- Interruption of the aorta, which can occur at three levels:
  - Type A: after left subclavian artery (Fig. 3.12c).
  - Type B: after left common carotid (Fig. 3.12a).
  - Type C: after brachiocephalic trunk (Fig. 3.12b).
- Almost always accompanied by a VSD with posterior deviation of the outlet septum causing a narrowed LVOT.

Associations

- Can be present in context of common arterial trunk.
- Bicuspid aortic valve may be present.
- 50% associated with 22q11 deletion (see p. 177).

Physiology

- The ascending aorta supplies the vessels prior to the interruption, and the arterial duct supplies vessels distal to the interruption.
- As PVR falls, there will be increased pulmonary blood flow through the duct and VSD leading to breathlessness.
- As the PDA closes, there will be disruption to the blood supply distal to the narrowing causing liver, kidney, and gut dysfunction and then shock.
- The posterior deviation of the outlet septum causes varying degrees of LVOTO.

Clinical features

- With the PDA open, lower limb saturations will be lower than right arm saturations (as long as there is normal branching of head and neck vessels) and BP will be similar.
- As the PDA closes, there will be an increasing BP gradient between the right arm and legs with reduced/absent femoral pulses.
- Infants will become increasingly breathless with signs of liver, kidney, and gut dysfunction and shock.
- There may or may not be a murmur.

Treatment

- Prostaglandin infusion is required to maintain the arterial duct.
- Most cases undergo primary repair with arch reconstruction and VSD closure in one operation.
- In cases of prematurity/low birth weight, bilateral PA banding and maintenance of prostaglandin infusion or ductal stent to allow growth for primary repair later.
- In some cases, repair can be staged, with arch repair and main pulmonary artery (MPA) band and then VSD closure at a later date.
- Yasui procedure: in some patients with severe LVOTO, the aorta may be anastomosed to the PA (Damus–Kaye–Stansel (DKS) anastomosis) with the VSD closed so that both leave the LV. A RV-to-PA shunt is then placed.

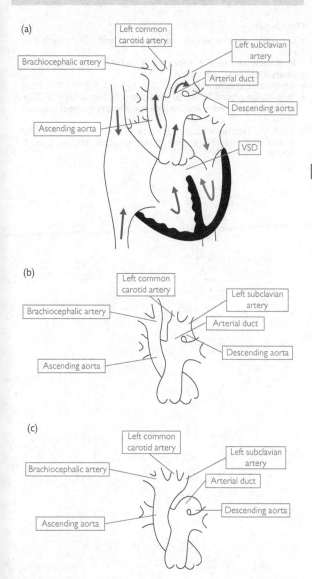

Fig. 3.12 Classification of interrupted aortic arch: (a) type B; (b) type C; (c) type A.

Outcomes
- Good postoperative survival rate, but with at least 35% reintervention rate.
- Most common area of reintervention is the LVOT, with subaortic obstruction requiring resection.
- Aortic valve replacement for AS.
- Ross–Konno procedure may be needed later to augment the LVOT and replace the aortic valve with the patient's pulmonary valve (homograft to the pulmonary position).
- If the Yasui procedure has been undertaken then the RV-to-PA conduit may need reintervention and will need replacement, although timing is variable.

Laterality disorders

Anatomy

- The thoracic and abdominal organs are not normally symmetrically arranged and there is a complex signalling process which leads to the final position of these organs during development.
- When the correct position and sidedness (laterality) of these organs is not achieved, it is referred to as a laterality disorder.
- The description is often referred to according to the pattern of the atrial appendages, as these are the most consistent indicators of the morphology of the atriums.
- Other terms used include visceral heterotaxy, Ivemark syndrome, or asplenia/polysplenia syndromes.
- *LA isomerism:*
  - Both atrial appendages are of LA morphology.
  - Primary feature is of interrupted IVC with azygous/hemiazygous continuity.
  - Ipsilateral pulmonary venous drainage or to the left-sided atrium.
  - Apex of the heart may be leftward deviated or pointing to the right.
  - *Can be* associated with major CHD.
- *RA isomerism:*
  - Both atrial appendages are of RA morphology.
  - IVC present but lies on same side as the aorta.
  - Cardiac apex may be to the right, left, or midline.
  - Bilateral SVCs are common.
  - Total anomalous pulmonary venous drainage (TAPVD) is present.
  - Major CHD *almost invariable*.

Associations

- Can be familial, although not commonly associated with chromosomal abnormalities.

Physiology

- This is defined by the systemic and pulmonary venous drainage and associated cardiac lesions.

Clinical features

- *LA isomerism:*
  - Can be asymptomatic if no associated CHD.
  - Associated with complete heart block or sinus bradycardia.
  - Abdominal associations:
    - Midline liver.
    - Malrotation of the intestines.
    - Duodenal or jejunal atresia.
    - Polysplenia (common) or asplenia (rare).
    - Biliary atresia (2%).
- *RA isomerism:*
  - Depends on associated CHD lesions which are very common.
  - Abdominal associations:
    - Midline/left liver.
    - Stomach on the right/opposite side to the heart.

- ○ Malrotation of the intestines.
- ○ Asplenia.

Treatment

- Treatment is not required for interrupted IVC alone, but associated CHD may require medical/surgical treatment.
- Surgical strategy depends on type of CHD and whether a 'corrective' strategy is feasible or if a single-ventricle strategy (Fontan) is required.
- Extracardiac findings may require specialist input, such as prophylactic penicillin for asplenia, abdominal surgery for malrotation/volvulus, and Kasai portoenterostomy for biliary atresia.

Outcomes

- Long-term outcome and quality of life depends on associated malformations.

Mitral stenosis

Anatomy

(See Fig. 3.13.)
- The normal mitral valve is bileaflet, composed of an anterior and posterior leaflet. The anterior leaflet is the larger of the two.
- Cords attach from each leaflet to two papillary muscles and help prevent regurgitation during systole.
- Congenital stenosis can be caused by:
  - A membrane just above the annulus restricting flow (supramitral membrane)
  - A small valve annulus
  - Reduced leaflet excursion from fusion of commissures
  - Short or thickened cords restricting leaflet motion
  - A single papillary muscle (parachute valve) restricting leaflet opening.
- Acquired stenosis from rheumatic heart disease is the most common form worldwide. It leads to thickening of the valve leaflets and apparatus.

Associations

- Associated with other left heart lesions including HLHS and Shone complex.

Physiology

- As the narrowing progresses, the transmitral gradient increases, leading to LA dilatation.
- Pulmonary venous congestion and pulmonary hypertension can ensue.
- In severe cases right heart failure can develop, with reduced cardiac output.

Clinical features

- Dyspnoea and reduced exercise tolerance.

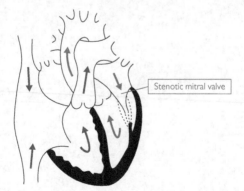

Stenotic mitral valve

Fig. 3.13 Mitral stenosis.

- Chronic cough from the enlarged LA compressing the left main bronchus.
- Signs of right heart failure in severe mitral stenosis.
- Diastolic murmur at the apex.
- Large LA can cause atrial arrhythmias.

Treatment

- Severe stenosis will require surgery to relieve the narrowing and repair the valve.
- Severely diseased valves may require a surgical valve replacement with a prosthetic valve (difficult in smaller patients).

Outcomes

- Dependent on the cause and severity of the disease.
- Severe untreated disease will result in death in the first few years of life.

Partial anomalous pulmonary venous drainage (PAPVD)

Anatomy

(See Fig. 3.14.)

- Usually, four pulmonary veins connect and drain oxygenated blood back to the LA.
- In PAPVD, one or more (but not all) veins connect anomalously.
- Typical drainage locations include the SVC or innominate vein, to the RA, or to the IVC.

Associations

- Frequently found in association with an ASD (especially sinus venosus type).

Physiology

- The effects of PAPVD are to divert pulmonary venous return to the right side resulting in increased Qp. This is physiologically similar to the effects of an ASD.

Clinical features

- PAPVD may go unnoticed for many years and present incidentally, this is in contrast to TAPVD which usually presents acutely in infancy.
- Clinical features depend on the number and size of the anomalous veins, the presence of an additional ASD, and the total size of the left-to-right shunt.
- Patients will frequently be asymptomatic.
- In those with high Qp, frequent chest infections can be common.
- Patients have normal saturations.
- Fixed splitting of the second heart sound or 'flow' murmur from relative pulmonary valve stenosis may be auscultated.

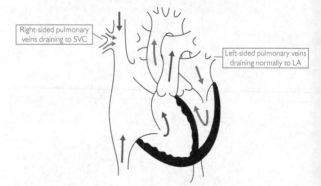

Right-sided pulmonary veins draining to SVC

Left-sided pulmonary veins draining normally to LA

Fig. 3.14 PAPVD.

Treatment

- A single small vein may be managed conservatively.
- Larger shunts particularly with a coexistent ASD may require intervention.
- Veins can be surgically baffled via the ASD to the LA.
- In older patients a stent can be used to baffle SVC flow into the RA and direct venous flow across the ASD into the LA.
- The Warden procedure can be used (see p. 130).

Outcomes

- Long-term outcomes following surgical repair are excellent unless the anatomy makes a more complex repair necessary.

Patent arterial duct (patent ductus arteriosus (PDA))

Anatomy

(See Fig. 3.15.)

- The arterial duct (ductus arteriosus) exists in fetal life to allow blood to bypass the lungs.
- Following birth, increased oxygenation, separation from the placenta, and loss of maternal prostaglandins usually cause the duct to constrict and then close within the first 72 hours of life.
- Persistence beyond this stage is known as a PDA.

Associations

- The incidence is inversely proportional to gestational age and weight.
- In preterm infants, 20–60% may have a PDA (80% of infants weighing <1200 g compared to 40% weighing 2000 g at birth).
- Other rare causes include congenital rubella and some genetic conditions.

Physiology

- As PVR falls after birth, the duct allows increased blood flow from the systemic to pulmonary circulation.
- Large ducts can allow significant increases in pulmonary blood flow and consequently decreased systemic perfusion.

Clinical features

- Clinical severity depends on the size of the duct.
- A continuous murmur is often heard.
- Bounding pulses due to low diastolic pressure.
- Increased work of breathing and failure to thrive may occur due to high Qp.

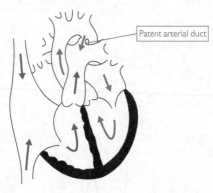

Patent arterial duct

Fig. 3.15 PDA.

- Reduced systemic blood flow may affect gut perfusion (risk factor for necrotizing enterocolitis in premature neonates especially if reversed flow in the mesenteric vessels), and renal perfusion.

Treatment

- Asymptomatic children are frequently reviewed at 1 year of age to allow time for the duct to close spontaneously.
- 'Silent' small ducts can be managed conservatively and may not require follow-up after 1-year review.
- Haemodynamically significant ducts can be treated medically (in neonates): ibuprofen, paracetamol, or indomethacin can be used to inhibit prostaglandins and encourage ductal closure.
- Interventional approaches include using small devices or coils to occlude the duct.
- Surgical ligation via a lateral thoracotomy may be performed, most commonly in very small infants.
- In patients with ducts demonstrating bidirectional flow, PVR should be assessed prior to intervention.

Outcomes

- Excellent results from interventional and surgical approaches.

Pulmonary atresia with intact ventricular septum/critical pulmonary stenosis

Anatomy

(See Fig. 3.16.)
- Critical narrowing or complete atresia of the pulmonary valve.
- May be associated with a varying size and morphology of the RV, PA, and tricuspid valve.
- May be associated with coronary sinusoids, where a coronary artery (usually right) is perfused retrogradely through channels from the high-pressure RV.

Associations

- Usually isolated but can be associated with genetic diseases in ~5%.

Physiology

- There is right-to-left shunting across the atrial septum causing cyanosis.
- Pulmonary blood supply is via the arterial duct.

Clinical features

- Usually presents in the first days of life due to cyanosis.
- Murmur (variable, depends on patency of pulmonary valve).

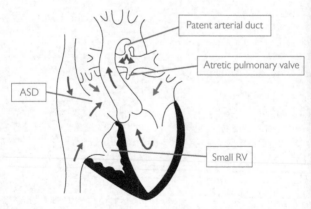

Fig. 3.16 Pulmonary atresia with intact ventricular septum.

Treatment

- Depends on the size of the RV.
- If tripartite/apex-forming then biventricular strategy is usually attempted, often via a catheter-based approach—radiofrequency perforation and balloon dilatation of the pulmonary valve.
- If coronary sinusoids are present, then relief of the valvar obstruction is usually not possible and therefore a single-ventricle strategy is required.
- If the RV is hypoplastic then additional procedures may be needed to improve pulmonary blood flow such as ductal stenting, a BTT shunt, or a Glenn shunt.
- Reintervention at a later point is almost inevitable to replace the pulmonary valve with a competent valve after balloon dilatation.

Outcomes

- Long-term outcome depends on treatment strategy (i.e. biventricular or single-ventricle circulation).
- Poor survival when coronary sinusoids are present.

Pulmonary atresia with ventricular septal defect

Anatomy

(See Fig. 3.17.)
* Sometimes also referred to as tetralogy of Fallot with pulmonary atresia.
* The aorta arises above a VSD, and this is the only outlet from the heart.
* The aortic arch is right sided in 30% of cases.
* The anatomy of the pulmonary vasculature is highly variable. The size of the PA ranges from absent through to well-developed, confluent branch PAs supplied by an arterial duct.
* In severe cases the native PAs are severely hypoplastic or absent and supplied by major aortopulmonary collateral arteries (MAPCAs).

Associations

* The commonest genetic association is the 22q11 deletion but may occur as part of the VACTERL association (see p. 183) and other syndromes.

Physiology

* The aorta receives a mixture of oxygenated and deoxygenated blood.
* Blood flow to the lungs is via the arterial duct or collateral vessels.
* Oxygen saturations are determined by pulmonary blood flow: high Qp results in high oxygen saturations (>90%) and low Qp in low saturations.

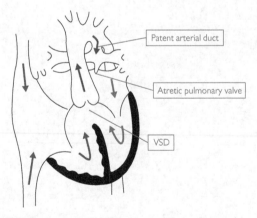

Patent arterial duct

Atretic pulmonary valve

VSD

Fig. 3.17 Pulmonary atresia with VSD.

Clinical features

- Cyanosis may be evident in the neonatal period. This will become severe as the duct constricts.
- A minority of infants may present with breathlessness and failure to thrive due to high Qp.

Treatment

- Surgical repair ideally includes closure of the VSD and insertion of a conduit between the RV and PAs.
- This depends on adequate development of pulmonary vascular bed. Insertion of a BTT shunt or a conduit between the RV and PAs may be required in advance of full repair.
- In complex cases, unifocalization of MAPCAs ± hypoplastic native PAs may be required in a staged fashion.
- A minority of cases may not be amenable to repair.

Outcome

- If pulmonary vascular anatomy permits full repair then outcome is favourable, although serial RV–PA conduit replacement or percutaneous valve implantation is required.
- Outcome is more guarded for complex cases with hypoplastic PAs and MAPCAs, in some cases there is no surgical option available.

Pulmonary stenosis (PS)

Anatomy

(See Fig. 3.18.)
- Narrowing of the pulmonary valve annulus (80% of cases), or subvalvar/supravalvar area.
- The valve is frequently thickened and may dome in systole and is often bicuspid or occasionally unicuspid.
- In infants the valve annulus, MPA, and branch PAs may also be hypoplastic.
- Narrowing of subvalvar area due to RV hypertrophy and thickining of septomarginal bands.

Associations

- Can be associated with genetic disorders including Noonan syndrome, Alagille syndrome, and Williams syndrome (see pp. 178–181).

Physiology

- There is obstruction to the outflow of blood from the RV, leading to RV pressure loading and right ventricular hypertrophy (RVH).
- In critical stenosis, the pulmonary blood flow will be duct dependent.
- As RVH develops, the RV becomes less compliant and diastolic dysfunction may occur.

Clinical features

- Related to the degree of obstruction but mild and moderate PS is well tolerated.
- In critical PS, pulmonary blood flow is insufficient leading to hypoxaemia, cyanosis, shock, and later to death.
- Severe PS can lead to dyspnoea, exercise intolerance, and hypoxaemia. High CVP can lead to hepatomegaly and oedema.

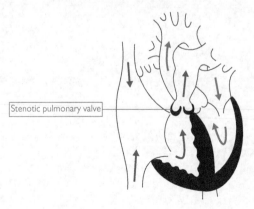

Stenotic pulmonary valve

Fig. 3.18 PS.

- Moderate PS presents with louder harsh murmur ± thrill and leads to RVH and a hyperdynamic precordium.
- Mild PS presents with a soft ejection systolic murmur at the upper left sternal edge radiating to the back or upper right sternal edge.

Treatment

- Mild or moderate PS can be managed conservatively.
- Severe stenosis requires relief from either an intervention or surgery depending on the underlying anatomy.
- Cardiac catheterization with balloon valvuloplasty can be effective for valvar stenosis.
- The presence of subvalvar or supravalvar stenosis may require surgical relief with augmentation of the hypoplastic vessel.

Outcomes

- Catheter-based approaches are typically safe and result in relief of the stenosis, with good long-term outcomes.
- Complications can include tearing of a leaflet and development of pulmonary valvar regurgitation.
- Serial follow-up imaging is required to monitor for recurrence of stenosis or to monitor the degree and effects of regurgitation.

Pulmonary vein stenosis

Anatomy

- Can either involve diffuse pulmonary vein hypoplasia, or discrete narrowing of pulmonary veins.

Associations

- More common in infants born prematurely (reasons unclear).
- Pulmonary vein stenosis can be seen after TAPVD repair in around 10% of cases.

Physiology

- Blood cannot flow freely back from the lungs leading to pulmonary congestion and elevation of right heart pressures.
- In presence of single-vein stenosis, there may be collateralization.

Clinical features

- Dependent on number and extent of veins involved.
- Diffuse pulmonary vein hypoplasia or atresia can present immediately after birth with profound desaturation.
- Discrete stenosis of a single vein may have minimal symptoms as there may be collateralization to the other vein on that side.
- More widespread stenosis presents with pulmonary congestion and respiratory symptoms with eventual elevation of right heart pressures.

Treatment

- Single vein involvement with minimal effect/collateralization may not need any treatment.
- Interventions may set up further inflammation and fibrosis leading to worsening sclerosis, and for this reason are often avoided.
- Surgery: in some cases there may be an identifiable surgical lesion which can be opened up using a 'sutureless' approach.
- Catheter: balloon dilatation or stenting of the pulmonary veins, recurrent procedures may be required.
- Chemotherapy: some centres advocate chemotherapy agents to try and reduce the inflammatory process, may be used in combination with approaches as above.
- Given the poor prognosis, particularly in the ex-premature infant with comorbidities or those with bilateral involvement in single-ventricle physiology, a non-intervention approach with palliative care involvement may be most appropriate.

Outcomes

- Congenital severe pulmonary vein hypoplasia and atresia has a very poor prognosis and is usually fatal in the neonatal period.
- Overall pulmonary vein stenosis mortality around 50%.
- Discrete stenosis may be ameliorated with surgery or a catheter procedure but reintervention rates high.

Systemic venous abnormalities

Anatomy

(See Fig. 3.19.)
- The two most common systemic venous abnormalities are interrupted IVC, and persistent left SVC.
- In interrupted IVC, there is usually azygous continuation to the SVC and eventually right heart.
- In persistent left SVC, drainage of this vessel is usually to the coronary sinus, so deoxygenated blood eventually drains to the RA.
- Drainage of the left SVC is rarely to the LA, or unroofed coronary sinus, causing systemic desaturation.
- Bilateral SVCs are more common than isolated left SVC.

Associations

- Anomalies of systemic venous drainage can occur alone, with other venous abnormalities, or with major CHD.
- Commonly seen in disorders of laterality (see p. 62).
- Left SVC is a common variant of normal, seen in 1:200 people.

Clinical findings

- Both interrupted IVC with azygous continuation and left SVC to coronary sinus can be asymptomatic if no associated CHD.
- Left SVC to LA or to unroofed coronary sinus will result in systemic desaturation.

Treatment

- Not usually required for these lesions alone, but may be required for associated CHD lesions.

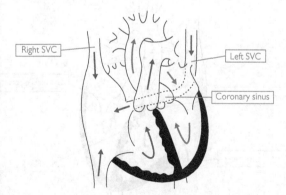

Fig. 3.19 Systemic venous abnormality: bilateral SVCs.

Tetralogy of Fallot

Anatomy

(See Fig. 3.20.)
- The primary abnormality is anterosuperior deviation of the infundibular septum which results in:
  - Large perimembranous VSD
  - Aorta overriding the crest of the ventricular septum
  - RVOTO/PS (varies from mild obstruction to atresia)
  - Secondary RVH.
- Additional valvular, supravalvular, and/or branch PA stenosis may be present.
- Aortic arch right sided in 30%.
- Associated with other CHDs, e.g. PDA, ASD, AVSD, and others.
- Tetralogy of Fallot with absent pulmonary valve is associated with absence of the arterial duct and dilated branch PAs which can cause airway compression/bronchomalacia.

Associations

- Highly associated with extracardiac and genetic abnormalities, most commonly trisomy 21 and 22q11 deletion (see p. 175 and p. 177).
- CHARGE, VACTERL, or Alagille syndrome may be present (see pp. 180–183).

Physiology

- Depends on the degree of RVOTO.
- If little/no RVOTO (less common) then left-to-right shunt akin to VSD with normal/near-normal oxygen saturations.

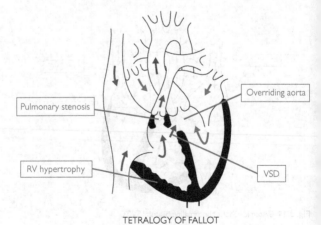

TETRALOGY OF FALLOT

Fig. 3.20 Tetralogy of Fallot.

- More severe RVOTO leads to decrease pulmonary blood flow and decreased oxygen saturations due to right-to-left shunt across the VSD.
- Branch PAs may be hypoplastic, depending on pulmonary blood flow.

Clinical features

- While the arterial duct is patent (or only mild obstruction to pulmonary blood flow), cyanosis may be absent.
- Minority have pulmonary over-circulation due to unobstructed left-to-right flow across the VSD.
- Oxygen saturations will vary with feeding and intercurrent illness.
- Hypercyanotic spells (see p. 314) may occur in infancy but 'squatting' very rare in modern practice due to repair in infancy.
- Finger clubbing, polycythaemia, and cerebral abscess may occur in unrepaired cases in childhood/adulthood.
- Systolic murmur (variable degree, but usually harsh) at the left upper sternal border, single second heart sound.

Treatment

- Initial management to maintain adequate oxygen saturations (>80%) following ductal closure. In most cases, primary surgical in infancy, typically around 6 months of age.
- If early severe cyanosis or cases of severe hypoxia in neonate, then BTT shunt or right ventricular outflow tract (RVOT) stent to increase the blood flow until surgical repair.
- Medical treatment with beta-blocker (e.g. propranolol for cyanotic spells). Emergency treatment (see p. 314) with oxygen, knee-to-chest position, and vasoconstrictors rarely required given the earlier surgery.

Outcomes

- Excellent postsurgical survival if no associated lesions.
- High chance of PA valve replacement later in life owing to pulmonary regurgitation causing progressive RV dilation/dysfunction.
- Lifelong follow-up required for cardiac function, RV volume, arrhythmia, branch PA stenosis, and aortic dilation.

Total anomalous pulmonary venous drainage (TAPVD)

Anatomy

(See Fig. 3.21.)

- All four pulmonary veins drain into a confluence and from there to the
  systemic venous system with variability in connection and in degree of
  obstruction:
  - *Supracardiac*: pulmonary veins drain into the brachiocephalic vein, to
    the right or left SVC or to the azygous vein (Fig. 3.21a).

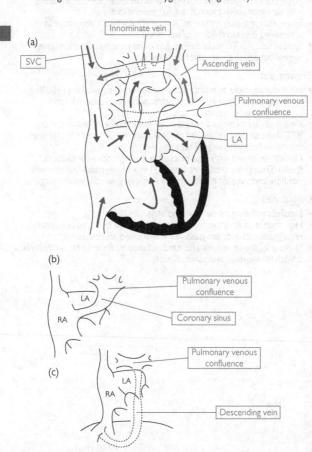

Fig. 3.21 TAPVD. (a) Supracardiac, (b) intracardiac, and (c) infracardiac types.

- *Intracardiac*: pulmonary veins drain into the coronary sinus or directly into the RA (in right isomerism) (Fig. 3.21b).
- *Infracardiac*: pulmonary veins drain to the portal vein or the venous duct via descending vein (Fig. 3.21c).
- Anomalous pulmonary venous drainage is part of laterality disorders, RA isomerism in particular.

Associations

- Isolated TAPVD is associated with an ASD, a VSD can also be present. It can be found in tetralogy of Fallot, HLHS, or common arterial trunk.
- Low association with extracardiac and genetic abnormalities (about 4%), including 'Cat eye' syndrome and Holt–Oram syndrome (see p. 182).

Physiology

- Since all pulmonary venous blood returns to the RA, saturations depend on the degree of mixing permitted by the size of the interatrial communication and degree of pulmonary venous obstruction.
- In cases of restrictive interatrial communication, there is limited blood flow reaching the LA reducing systemic output.
- Since both systemic and pulmonary venous blood return to the RA, the RA pressure rises causing congestion in both the systemic and pulmonary circuits.
- Secondary PA hypertension may occur in the setting of pulmonary venous obstruction. The site of obstruction is usually in the vein draining the pulmonary venous confluence.

Clinical features

- Rapid deterioration in the first day of life in those with obstructed TAPVD, with progressive dyspnoea, feeding difficulties, cardiorespiratory failure, severe respiratory distress, hypoxia, and acidosis.
- Slower development of cardiorespiratory failure in those with unobstructed TAPVD.
- Loud first heart sound, fixed split second sound with accentuated pulmonary component.
- Soft systolic murmur may be present as well as venous hum.

Treatment

- Surgical treatment performed as soon as possible after clinical state is optimized.
- Obstructed TAPVD is a surgical emergency and one of the few reasons to operate on CHD out of hours.
- This involves reconnection of the pulmonary veins to the LA.

Outcomes

- 95% 30-day postoperative survival in the UK with overall good outcome except in those with infracardiac form of TAPVD where there is pulmonary venous obstruction.
- In patients with associated RA isomerism the outcome is very poor.
- In a minority of patients reintervention to the pulmonary veins is necessary due to recurrent progressive obstruction which can be extremely difficult to manage.

Transposition of the great arteries (TGA)

Anatomy

(See Fig. 3.22.)
- There is atrioventricular (AV) concordance and ventriculoarterial (VA) discordance, so that the aorta arises from the RV and PA from the LV.
- Can be so-called simple TGA, or combined with various other lesions, commonly:
  - VSDs
  - LVOTO/PS.
- Most often seen with usual atrial arrangement but can also be seen with mirror-image arrangement of the atria.
- The aortic valve often has a complete muscular infundibulum, and the pulmonary valve leaflets are in fibrous continuity with the mitral valve.
- The coronary arteries arise from the aorta in a variety of patterns.

Associations

- Not commonly associated with genetic or chromosomal syndromes.

Physiology

- The systemic and pulmonary circulations are in parallel, rather than in series as in the normal anatomy.
- Without any communication between the two parallel circulations, the systemic circulation would rapidly desaturate, and death would ensue.
- Communications are possible at the level of the arterial duct and atrial septum, and at ventricular level if a VSD is present.

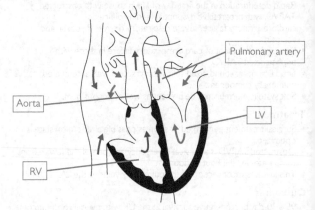

Fig. 3.22 Transposition of the great arteries.

- The direction and amount of blood flow at these points is variable and is dependent on the size of the communication and the PVR.
- Immediately after birth the PVR is high and flow at the PDA is bidirectional, or even right to left (PA to aorta). As PVR falls, the blood flow through the PDA will become left to right (aorta to PA), increasing pulmonary blood flow, pulmonary venous return, and thus left-to-right flow at atrial level.

Clinical features

- At birth there will be a variable degree of cyanosis, depending on the degree of mixing between the two circulations.
- If the atrial communication is restrictive may immediately present with extreme cyanosis and shock.
- So-called reversed differential cyanosis is pathognomonic of TGA (due to PDA flow from the PA to the aorta) producing postductal saturations that are higher than preductal.
- Second heart sound may be single.
- May be other clinical signs of associated lesions (e.g. a murmur from a VSD).

Treatment

- An infusion of prostaglandin should be commenced to ensure ductal patency.
- Consider the need for balloon atrial septostomy (BAS; see p. 168).
- Treat acidosis and hypovolaemia with volume replacement.
- Oxygen may be helpful to lower PVR.
- Plan for surgical management—in the majority of cases an arterial switch operation can be performed (see p. 137), usually performed at between 7 and 14 days of life.
- An arterial switch operation may be precluded by associated lesions (e.g. severe LVOTO or an adverse coronary arrangement), in which case an alternative surgical strategy will be required.

Outcomes

- Excellent short-term surgical survival.
- Excellent long-term survival, although some require further intervention to the branch PAs, or coronary arteries.
- Some evidence that there is an increased risk of pulmonary hypertension, and subtle neurodevelopmental disorders in later childhood.

Tricuspid atresia

Anatomy

(See Fig. 3.23.)
- Describes 'absent right AV connection', i.e. complete absence of the tricuspid valve (with atrial floor separated from RV by fibrofatty AV groove) and no inflow portion of RV. True 'atresia' of the tricuspid valve with an imperforate membrane is extremely rare.
- A VSD is almost always present.
- The great arteries are normally related in 70% (usually with PS).
- The great arteries are transposed in 30% (sometimes with AS/coarctation of the aorta/interrupted aortic arch).

Associations

- Usually isolated, although associations have been described with trisomy 18 and VACTERL (see p. 174 and p. 183).

Physiology

- Obligate right-to-left shunt at atrial level.
- Blood flow into the RV is through the VSD.
- The size of VSD may influence pulmonary blood flow/size of branch PAs (if arteries are normally related) or systemic blood flow/aortic development (if arteries are transposed).
- VSD may become more restrictive over time.

Clinical features

- Cyanosis is usually severe from birth.
- May be history of hypoxic spells if substrate for sub-PS.
- Single second heart sound with 2–3/6 holosystolic or early systolic murmur VSD at lower left sternal edge.
- Continuous murmur of PDA.
- Hepatomegaly if high venous pressures/restrictive atrial septum.

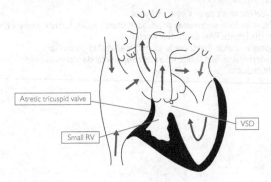

Atretic tricuspid valve

VSD

Small RV

Fig. 3.23 Tricuspid atresia.

Treatment

- BAS may be needed if restrictive atrial septum.
- Initial surgical strategy depends on pulmonary blood flow and relationship of great vessels (either to augment or reduce pulmonary blood flow, if needed).
- All patients will ultimately require single-ventricle palliation.

Outcomes

- Long-term outcome mainly determined by single-ventricle physiology.
- Specific data for tricuspid atresia: survival 90% at 1 month, 81% at 1 year, 70% at 10 years, and 60% at 20 years.

Vascular rings and slings

Anatomy

(See Fig. 3.24.)

- A vascular *ring* is an anatomical arrangement where vascular structures completely encircle the trachea and oesophagus. Double aortic arch and right aortic arch with left arterial duct are the most common.
- A vascular *sling* is when vascular structures cause a partial ring around the trachea and/or oesophagus. Examples include a left PA sling or a left aortic arch with an aberrant right subclavian artery.

Associations

- Vascular rings can coexist with CHD (e.g. tetralogy of Fallot, AVSD, VSD), and genetic/chromosomal abnormalities such as microdeletion of chromosome 22q11.2 and trisomy 21 (see pp. 175–177).
- A left PA sling can occur with complete tracheal rings and other abnormalities of the tracheal anatomy.

Clinical features

- Not all patients are symptomatic in infancy.
- Features which may be apparent include:
  - Noisy breathing
  - Stridor—typically expiratory, but can be inspiratory or biphasic
  - Respiratory distress
  - Recurrent lower respiratory tract infections
  - Dysphagia/choking with solid foods
  - Exertional asthma/wheeze
  - Difficult-to-control 'asthma'.
- Due to nature of symptoms, patients may present to primary care, general paediatrics, ear, nose, and throat (ENT), or respiratory physicians.
- If respiratory symptoms are present, investigation is with bronchoscopy and/or computed tomography (CT) scan. Note that arterial ductal ligaments/atretic segments of aortic arches will not be visible on contrast-enhanced CT.

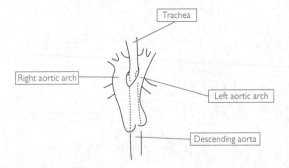

Fig. 3.24 Vascular ring: double aortic arch.

- If dysphagia is the predominant feature, investigation can be with barium swallow or video fluoroscopy and involvement of speech and language therapists and dietetic support.
- Investigation and treatment should be discussed on a case-by-case basis. Note that symptoms may not correlate with severity of tracheal compression. Careful history taking and multidisciplinary team (MDT) involvement is essential.

Treatment

- Surgery for vascular rings causing tracheobronchial compression:
  - Double aortic arch: ligate and divide both the smaller arch and the ductal ligament.
  - Right aortic arch with left arterial duct/ligament: division of the arterial ductal ligament. If aberrant in origin, the left subclavian artery may also need to be addressed by means of division/reimplantation/reduction/pexy.
- For left PA sling the left pulmonary is reimplanted into the MPA.
- An aberrant right subclavian artery can be divided if sufficient collateral supply to the right arm is present.

Outcomes

- Excellent outcomes following surgery.
- A proportion of patients with vascular rings may have ongoing respiratory symptoms postoperatively usually due to secondary tracheomalacia.
- Few require further surgery. Tracheostomy, aortopexy, or tracheopexy are rarely required as secondary treatments.

Ventricular septal defect (VSD)

Anatomy

(See Fig. 3.25.)
- Defined as a communication between the ventricles.
- Vary in size, number, shape, and location.
- Classified by their location within the ventricular septum and their borders as viewed from the RV:
  - *Perimembranous*: most common, involves the thin fibrous portion of the ventricular septum at the crux characterized by continuity of the tricuspid and aortic valves and can extend towards the inlet or outlet portion of the septum.
  - *Muscular*: has entirely muscular borders, and can occur in the inlet, outlet, or trabecular portions of the septum.
  - *Doubly committed subarterial*: located in the outlet portion of the septum, with fibrous continuity of the aortic and pulmonary valves.

Associations

- May be isolated, associated with other CHD, or as part of a more complex lesion (e.g. tetralogy of Fallot).

Physiology

- Flow across a VSD is dependent on the balance of SVR:PVR and the size of the defect.
- At birth, PVR is high and flow may be bidirectional or right to left.
- As PVR falls there will be increasing pulmonary blood flow with normal saturations and volume loading of the LV.
- Haemodynamically significant shunts with a high Qp tend to present once the PVR falls (around 6–8 weeks of age).
- Restrictive VSDs are those with a small shunt of no haemodynamic significance.
- With a large, unrestrictive VSDs, pulmonary hypertension is invariable if left untreated.

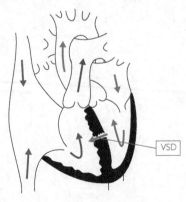

Fig. 3.25 VSD.

Clinical features

- Clinical features depend on the size, position, and number of defects and their cumulative left-to-right shunt.
- Small defects may be asymptomatic and suspected due to murmur.
- Large shunts can cause clinical features of heart failure secondary to high pulmonary blood flow (see p. 12).
- A murmur may be detected at any age and may be louder in smaller defects.
- A pansystolic murmur localized to the lower left sternal edge is typical.

Treatment

- Small defects (often described as 'restrictive') are often asymptomatic and may be treated conservatively if there is a small shunt and no clinical signs of pulmonary over-circulation (spontaneous closure of perimembranous or small muscular VSDs is common).
- Large (or 'unrestrictive') defects result in high Qp and may require medical management with diuretics and feeding/respiratory support.
- For large defects, in most cases primary surgical closure is performed in the first 3–6 months of life. If surgically inaccessible then a PA band may be performed initially.
- Selected cases suitable for interventional device closure in older patients.
- Medium-sized defects require monitoring for signs of high pulmonary blood flow and pulmonary hypertension—the natural history is reduction of size.
- Coronary cusp prolapse (usually right coronary cusp) may cause aortic valve regurgitation for which surgery is indicated.

Outcomes

- Small VSDs can be managed conservatively.
- Very good long-term surgical outcomes.

Cardiac investigations in children

Introduction

Non-invasive imaging and physiological testing are used extensively in children with heart disease. Both may have utility in establishing the initial diagnosis, severity stratification, and serial monitoring. As imaging techniques have developed, we have seen magnetic resonance imaging (MRI) and CT largely replace invasive imaging techniques such as cardiac catheterization with angiography.

Both the acquisition and interpretation of images require specialized knowledge, so these investigations tend to be performed in centres with dedicated paediatric cardiac imaging services.

Chest X-ray (CXR)

Chest X-ray (CXR)

The CXR is a simple and easy-to-perform investigation which remains an important diagnostic tool in children with heart disease (Fig. 4.1). Adult films are usually taken with the patient standing in front of the film with the X-ray source behind them (posteroanterior (PA) film). In babies and usually in children, films are taken the other way round (anteroposterior (AP))—this magnifies the heart size.

From a cardiac perspective, the following should be assessed systematically:
- *Situs*: the gastric bubble is normally left-sided.
- *Diaphragm*: the right side is usually slightly higher. A raised hemidiaphragm may be caused by lung volume loss or phrenic nerve palsy (following cardiac surgery).
- *Heart position*: cardiac apex normally left, can be central or to the right.
- *Heart size*: the cardiothoracic ratio should be <0.5 unless AP projection.
- *Lung fields*: normal, oligaemic (may be due to reduced pulmonary blood flow, e.g. PS) or plethoric (may be due to excess pulmonary blood flow, e.g. in VSD or AVSD).
- *Costophrenic angles*: clear or evidence of pleural effusion.
- *Mediastinum*: normal, widened (e.g. aortic aneurysm), enlarged lymph nodes, thymic shadow in infants, or narrow pedicle (e.g. TGA).
- *Prosthetic devices*: e.g. duct occluders, ASD occluders, and coils.

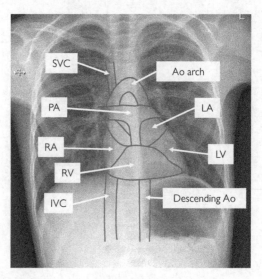

Fig. 4.1 CXR with cardiac contour drawn over. Ao, aorta.

Cardiac silhouette

Distinctive patterns are described with certain anomalies:
- In lesions with hypoplastic/absent MPA, a 'PA bay' may be seen.
- Tetralogy of Fallot: 'boot-shaped' heart with elevated apex.
- Ebstein's anomaly: 'wall-to-wall heart'.
- TGA: narrow mediastinal pedicle, 'egg on a string'.
- TAPVD: 'snowman sign'.

12-lead electrocardiogram (ECG)

The 12-lead ECG remains a first-line tool in the investigation of children with symptoms of, or confirmed, heart disease or arrhythmia.

Lead positioning

Standard lead positions are used (Fig. 4.2). In neonates and younger children, smaller electrodes are used. In active children, positioning the limb leads over more proximal bony structures (shoulder and hips) may reduce movement artefact compared with distal limb placements.

Standard settings

Initially use standard settings for speed (25 mm/sec) and amplitude (10 mm/mV). These are demonstrated in Fig. 4.3.

Basic principles of ECG interpretation

The interpretation of a 12-lead ECG in children must be approached systemically to avoid missing details not obvious on first review.

- *The clinical context*: understand the indication for ECG, e.g. a family history of sudden cardiac death (SCD) requires focus on signs of inherited channelopathies, such as the corrected QT interval.
- *The ECG settings*: confirming standard ECG settings and positions.
- *Overview*: before focusing on a systemic analysis of each lead and component in turn, the ECG can be reviewed as a whole, identifying any obvious abnormalities or irregularities in rhythm.

- A 'superior QRS axis' is from −30° to −180° and is always abnormal. It may be caused by CHD, e.g.:
  - AVSD
  - Tricuspid atresia.

- *Heart rate* (HR): each large square is 0.2 sec at standard settings. In a regular rhythm, HR equals 300 divided by the RR interval (measured in

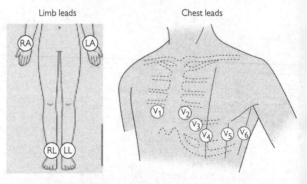

Fig. 4.2 Standard ECG lead position diagrams.

Limb leads

Chest leads

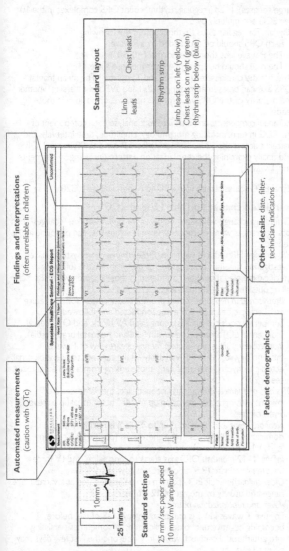

Automated measurements
(caution with QTc)

Findings and interpretations
(often unreliable in children)

Standard layout

Limb leads	Chest leads
Rhythm strip	

Limb leads on left (yellow)
Chest leads on right (green)
Rhythm strip below (blue)

Standard settings

25 mm/s

10mm*

25 mm/sec paper speed
10 mm/mV amplitude*

Other details: date, filter,
technician, indications

Patient demographics

Fig. 4.3 Normal ECG, labelled to show normal settings.

large squares). In an irregular rhythm, count QRS complexes in the 10 sec ECG and multiply by 6.

- *Rhythm*: for regular sinus rhythm confirm the following:
  - Each QRS should be proceeded by a P wave.
  - The P-wave axis should be normal (~0–90°).
  - The rate should be appropriate for the child's age.
- *Axis*: are the cardiac axes (P, QRS, and T) normal? The mean frontal QRS axis can be estimated using leads I and aVF and assessing whether the majority of the QRS waveform is negative, or positive in those leads.
- *Individual components and time intervals*: analyse each component of the ECG in turn, including morphology, amplitude, time intervals, and patterns across the 12 leads; moving from P wave to PR interval, QRS, and finally examining the repolarization pattern (including ST segments and T waves).

Normal ECG values can be found in the Appendix (see p. 320).

Age-related changes on the 12-lead ECG

ECG findings change with age. Below is an outline of key changes seen across age ranges with reference to normal values that can be found in the appendix.

- *HR*: average HR reduces with age. Other than a more systems-based investigation for sinus bradycardias or tachycardias, the following specific examples should be considered in those children with HRs falling outside of the normal ranges.
  - *Bradycardia in neonates* should prompt closer review for premature atrial ectopic beats (that are not conducted and followed by compensatory sinus pauses), congenital AV block, and QT interval (congenital LQTS can present with fetal and neonatal bradycardia).
  - *Inappropriate 'sinus' tachycardia for any age*: review of P-wave morphology, axis, and HR variability—take care not to overlook atrial ectopic tachycardias (particularly those arising from a high atrial focus, see p. 207).
- *QRS axis and forces*: during early neonatal life, the RV forces are dominant with right axis deviation up to 145° being usual up to several months of age:
  - *Neonate*: right axis deviation (up to +145°) is normal with a dominance of RV forces in the chest leads (positive R:S ratio in leads V1–3).
  - *Infant (1–12 months)*: QRS axis starts to 'normalize' and LV forces become dominant (R:S ratio increases towards V4–6).
  - *Older child*: the adult ECG pattern can be appreciated at a variable age range and usually by the age of 12–16 years.
- *T waves and repolarization pattern*:
  - Positive T waves in V1 is common on days 1–3 of life, before becoming negative until older childhood, or sometimes persisting into adulthood. Positive T waves in V1 beyond the first few days may point to RVH or strain.
  - Negative T waves are normal in V1–3 in infants and children, anticipating that in teenage years V2–3 often will become positive.

    Negative T waves extending to V4 or beyond should prompt further
    review and investigation.
- *Corrected QT interval* (QTc): accurate measurement and estimation
  of QTc can be challenging in neonates due to relatively flat T waves.
  The QTc in healthy neonates can be up to 440 ms and can prolong
  further in the first 10–14 days of life before decreasing. Pragmatically,
  mild prolongation (440–470 ms) of the QTc in neonatal life warrants a
  repeat ECG at 1–2 months of age.

Common normal variants in children

The following findings are normal but sometimes cause concern:
- *Sinus arrhythmia*: can be pronounced in young, active children and is a
  normal finding. The RR interval should change over several beats in a
  cyclical fashion related to respiratory variation. More pronounced, or
  sudden rate changes may warrant further review with a longer ECG
  rhythm strip to better characterise.
- *Low atrial rhythm*: this is a normal finding at lower rates and does not
  require any further investigation if isolated. It is manifested by inverted
  P waves in the inferior leads. If there is any question of sinus node
  dysfunction (symptoms, family history, etc.), a simple test can be to ask
  the child to exercise and demonstrating normal P waves at higher HRs.
- *Atrial premature beats*: particularly common in neonates, atrial
  premature beats are a common and largely benign finding. In neonates
  they may present with marked HR irregularity or bradycardia, due to
  non-conducted atrial ectopy and compensatory sinus pauses. They tend
  to improve with time and if seen in the first few days of life in a well
  neonate, require no other investigation other than a repeat ECG in 1–2
  months.
- *First-degree AV block*: relatively common in older children and usually a
  benign finding. Any positive history (i.e. syncope) or family history of
  conduction disease may warrant further investigation. In neonatal life
  (or following cardiac surgery), this does need further monitoring for
  progressive atrioventricular node (AVN) dysfunction.
- *Wenckebach (second-degree AV block, Mobitz type I)*: a common finding
  in older children, particularly sporty teenagers at rest (due to high vagal
  tone), or children of most ages at night (often reported as an incidental
  finding on ambulatory monitoring). Similar to first-degree AV block, it is
  usually a benign finding, but should be taken in clinical context.
- *RSR pattern in V1–2 leads*: a narrow complex QRS with an RSR pattern
  in V1–2 is a normal finding in children.

Ambulatory ECG

Ambulatory heart rhythm monitoring is an important tool in paediatric cardiology, with a variety of different types of monitor available.

Common indications include:

- Paroxysmal symptoms (e.g. palpitations or syncope)
- Monitoring for arrhythmia burden (e.g. asymptomatic arrhythmias or frequent ventricular ectopy)
- Measuring HR profile for medication effect and compliance, or in bradyarrhythmias such as congenital complete heart block
- Screening/asymptomatic monitoring in high-risk groups (e.g. Fontan circulation, inherited arrhythmia).

Types of monitors available:

- *24–48-hour Holter* (record three leads) ± symptom diary.
- *3-14 day Holter*: extended recording (older devices may be limited to one lead).
- Adhesive patch *extended continuous ambulatory rhythm monitors*: allow continuous, single-lead recordings up to 30 days (single use and some are water resistant for swimming).
- *External loop recorders*: record up to 30 days, continuous 'loop memory' with ability to automatically detect arrhythmias and other events ('event recorders').
- *Implantable loop recorders*: implanted under the skin for up to 3 years, recording automatically/on symptom activation.
- *Mobile/smartphone-based ECG device*: some now able to record six-lead ECGs.

Selection of device

The selection of the appropriate monitor for the patient depends on the age of the child and frequency of symptoms. In syncopal children, the symptom will typically be recorded *after* the event, therefore requiring a loop recorder (that can retrospectively save heart rhythms), or continuous recording and careful symptom labelling.

Exercise ECG

A 12-lead ECG during exercise can be helpful in eliciting arrhythmias not apparent on a baseline resting ECG. Children as young as 3–4 years old can manage the test, which is either performed on a treadmill or cycle ergometer with increasing workload while recording a continuous 12-lead ECG.

Indications

* *Symptoms on exercise*: can be helpful in evaluating children with histories of exercise-induced, or post-exertional symptoms, specifically palpitations, presyncope, or collapse. It has particularly poor *positive* diagnostic yield in children with chest pain and cannot be relied upon to evaluate ST-segment changes if coronary ischaemia (angina) is suspected (uncommon in children).
* *Ventricular ectopy on baseline ECG*: usually suppressed on higher HRs during exercise (reassuring); however, in a small percentage worsens on exercise prompting further evaluation and treatment.
* *CPVT* (see p. 212): both for screening of family members and to evaluate treatment response for patients on antiarrhythmic drugs.
* *Long QT* (see p. 218): helpful in diagnosis of LQTS (during 4th minute of recovery) and evaluating HR response on treatment.
* *ICDs*: in selected children with ICDs, exercise tests may help define HR profile on exercise in a controlled setting, to monitor or adjust antiarrhythmic medication, and avoid inappropriate sensing and treatment of sinus tachycardia by the device.
* Sports screening: pre-participation exercise stress tests in young athletes are recommended in some countries (not in the UK), with increased diagnostic yield (when performed in addition to resting ECG), at the expense of a higher rate of false positives.

Cardiopulmonary exercise testing (CPET)

CPET is a means of objective assessment of exercise tolerance (Box 4.1). It is of value in paediatric cardiology because:
- Routine investigations assess the patient in the resting state, thus lacking assessment of the underlying haemodynamics with exercise.
- Subjective assessments by patients or parents correlate poorly with objective CPET.
- Serial data enables objective assessment of response to treatment (e.g. pre- and post-pulmonary valve replacement).

Oxygen consumption must increase to sustain metabolism during exercise, producing increased carbon dioxide which must be eliminated by the lungs. When maximum oxygen supply is reached, anaerobic metabolism takes over producing more carbon dioxide, which needs to be eliminated by increased ventilation. The point of inflection where this occurs is referred to as the anaerobic threshold (AT).

A CPET study assesses the integrated relationship between:
- External respiration
- Cardiovascular function
- Metabolic processes.

Box 4.1 Key CPET metrics

Workload imposed during testing
- Measured in watts (W).
- Basic lung function and mechanics.
- Forced expiratory volume in the first second (FEV_1) and forced vital capacity (FVC).
- Tidal volume (VT), respiratory rate, minute ventilation (VE).
- Dead space (VD) ventilation (VD/VT).

Gas exchange parameters
- Arterial saturations (SaO_2).
- Carbon dioxide production (VCO_2).
- Oxygen uptake (VO_2).
- Inspired or expired oxygen concentrations (FiO_2, FEO_2).
- Respiratory exchange ratio (RER): the ratio of carbon dioxide elimination to oxygen uptake per unit time.
- Breathing reserve (BR): a marker of ventilatory limitation to exercise and is calculated from other measured respiratory parameters.
- Ventilatory equivalent (EqO_2, $EqCO_2$) are measures of the efficiency of ventilation.

Cardiac parameters
- BP.
- HR (+ stress ECG).
- Oxygen pulse (O_2 pulse): ratio of VO_2/HR as an index of stroke volume.

CPET protocol

Can be performed with a treadmill or cycle ergometer (minimum height 130 cm).

The workload (W) and rate of increase (W/min) are adjusted based on the patient's age, size, comorbidity, and patient-reported fitness level. The aim is to achieve peak performance without early exhaustion or prolonged submaximal work over a 10–14-minute test. This typically includes 3 minutes of loadless cycling, 6–8 minutes of increasing workload, and 3 minutes of active recovery.

The following are recorded throughout:
- Gas exchange (measured via face mask).
- Oxygen saturations.
- 12-lead ECG.
- Non-invasive BP.

CPET results

These are displayed in graphical form on a 'nine-panel plot' to facilitate assessment of specific components of the physiology. Key reporting goals are to:
- Determine the adequacy of the test in terms of maximal effort
- Analyse respiratory, cardiac, and metabolic parameters.

The test is considered reliable for full interpretation of gas exchange parameters only if AT is achieved, as some patients may stop before this point due to poor compliance with the test.
- *VO2 max* (maximal oxygen uptake): marker of how well oxygen can be delivered to muscles. Frequently used to define the extent of cardiac limitations. It is the point at which VO_2 plateaus despite an increase in work rate.
- *Peak VO2* is the highest VO_2 value achieved with exercise and may be lower than VO_2 max if the patient stops the test early.
- *Oxygen pulse* (VO_2/HR) slope is normally a linear dynamic relationship of HR to oxygen uptake and is an index of stroke volume. An early plateau and low maximal value are markers of impaired stroke volume.
- *Ventilatory equivalents* when increased, indicate increased dead space. The nadir of Ve/VCO_2 is when Ve increases to eliminate carbon dioxide in response to metabolic acidosis. A steep Ve/VCO_2 slope is a marker of ventilation:perfusion mismatch and is seen in conditions where pulmonary perfusion is not increased either due to poor cardiac function, mechanical obstruction, or pulmonary hypertension.

Determining coexisting respiratory and metabolic conditions in patients with cardiac disease can be possible by expert interpretation of the nine-panel plots.

Tilt testing

Head-up tilt-table testing can be helpful in evaluating children presenting with recurrent syncope, presyncope, or palpitations, where the diagnosis is suggestive of vasovagal syncope, but remains uncertain. Most units have their own protocol for testing, e.g.:

• A period of around 10–15 minutes supine
• Following by head-up tilt to 60–70° for up to 45 minutes.

Drugs, such as glyceryl trinitrate (GTN) can increase sensitivity, at the expense of reducing the specificity of the test. It is important to correlate any symptoms on the tilt table with those experienced clinically (both patient and observing parent) while monitoring HR and BP response, allowing discrimination of physiological cause of symptoms, namely:

• *Vasodepressor*: inappropriate peripheral vasodilation, hypotension, and subsequent cerebral hypoperfusion
• *Cardioinhibitory*: less common in children, where sudden drop in HR precedes symptoms and hypotension
• *Mixed response*: showing an inappropriate drop in both BP and HR prior to syncope/symptoms.

Clear documentation of the exact timing of syncope/symptoms during the tilt test is also key in determining ongoing treatment. For example, in a mixed response with both hypotension and bradycardia, a syncopal episode occurring at the point of hypotension, but prior to bradycardia or asystole is unlikely to respond to cardiac pacing.

Transthoracic echocardiography (TTE)

TTE is the most common imaging modality used for the diagnosis and follow-up of paediatric heart disease. It is a vital skill for all paediatric cardiologists (but it is beyond the scope of this handbook to provide full instruction).

A sequential segmental approach should be followed, allowing for every segment and connection to be carefully delineated. There are a large number of possible imaging planes, which are varied by moving both the position of the probe on the patient's body and angling the ultrasound beam in different directions.

Summary of key views

Some of the most important views are outlined in Fig. 4.4a–e, but there are many more possibilities.

Subcostal view—probe placed below the xiphisternum, probe marker to the patient's left

Apical view four-chamber view—probe placed at the cardiac apex, usually close to left fifth intercostal space, midclavicular line, probe marker to patient's left

Parasternal long-axis view (PLAX)—probe placed at left third intercostal space, adjacent to the sternum, probe position to patient's right shoulder

Parasternal short-axis (PSAX) view—probe placed at left third intercostal space, adjacent to the sternum, probe position to patient's left shoulder

Suprasternal aortic arch view—probe placed in suprasternal notch, probe marker to around 1 o'clock

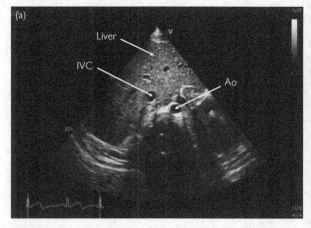

Fig 4.4 (Contd.)

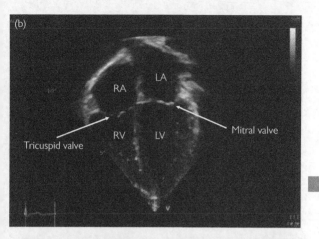

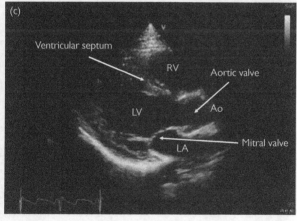

Fig 4.4 (Contd.)

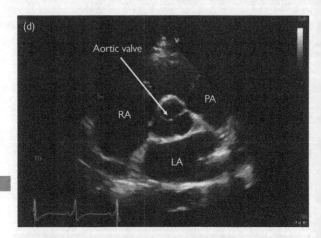

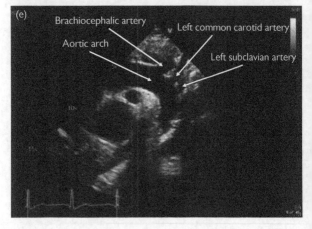

Fig. 4.4 (a) Labelled abdominal situs view. (b) Labelled apical four-chamber view. (c) Labelled PLAX view. (d) Labelled PSAX view. (e) Labelled arch view.

Other measurements and assessments

In addition to two-dimensional (2D) B-mode ultrasound images, additional haemodynamic and functional information can be obtained using more advanced techniques:

- *Spectral Doppler*: this allows the measurement of blood velocity. From velocity, pressure gradients can be estimated, using the modified Bernoulli equation:
  - Pressure difference (in mmHg) = $4 \times$ velocity^2 (in m/sec).
- *Colour Doppler*: this uses the Doppler technique to image the blood pool and demonstrate direction of flow (red = towards the probe, blue = away from the probe).
- *Tissue Doppler*: this uses the Doppler effect to measure the velocity and direction of myocardial movement, rather than blood. This is useful for the quantification of myocardial function.
- *M-mode*: this displays a single one-dimensional echo plane over time, also useful for assessing function.
- *Three-dimensional (3D) imaging*: requires specialist training and software but can be very useful for assessing and displaying spatial relationships between intracardiac structures and lesions.
- *Speckle-tracking*: this assesses myocardial motion and therefore function by automatically tracking the normal speckle pattern seen within the muscle.

Transoesophageal echocardiography (TOE)

TOE is used less frequently than TTE, because it is more invasive and usually requires a general anaesthetic (GA) in children. However, it has advantages of very high temporal and spatial resolution. The TOE probe is introduced into the oesophagus via the mouth or very occasionally via a nasal route. Care is required while introducing the probe to avoid potential complications.

Indications
- Routinely used perioperatively to assess the results of cardiac surgery and to monitor for complications.
- During catheter intervention, to guide placement of devices, visualize catheters/guidewires, and facilitate transseptal puncture.
- Sometimes used in the investigation of infectious endocarditis, as higher sensitivity to detect vegetations.

Potential complications (in addition to GA risk)
- Damage to teeth, pharynx, or oesophagus.
- Airway compression.
- Bleeding.
- Arrhythmia.

Contraindications
- Unrepaired oesophageal fistula.
- Oesophageal stricture.
- Uncontrolled gastrointestinal bleeding—particular caution is required in the presence of oesophageal varices.

Imaging technique
TOE probes have a number of controls to alter the plane of the ultrasound beam:
- Flexion/retroflexion.
- Rotational plane of the ultrasound beam from zero to 180°.
- By insertion/withdrawal of the probe, the plane can be changed through upper to mid to lower oesophagus.

Transgastric views are obtained by advancing the probe into the stomach and flexing it back to achieve different views such as short axis of the AV valves.

Summary of key views
A selection of key TOE views are shown in Fig. 4.5a–e:

Four-chamber view 120° view

45° view

Atrial septal view

Transgastric view

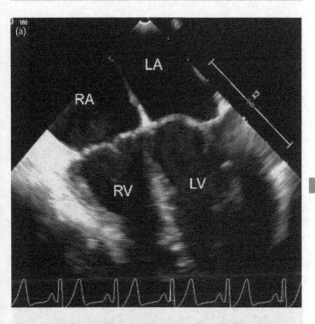

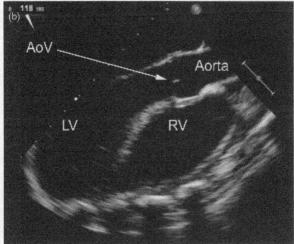

Fig 4.5 (*Contd.*)

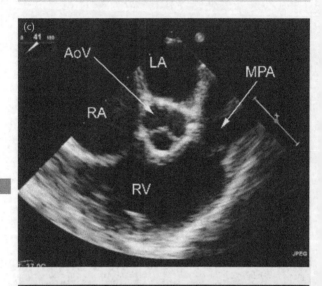

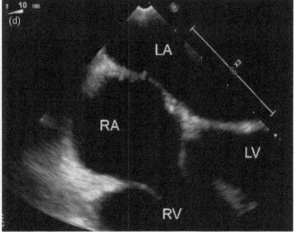

Fig 4.5 (*Contd.*)

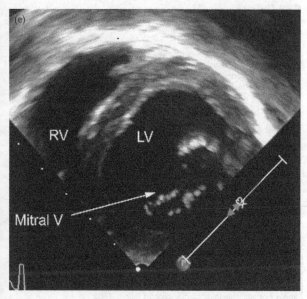

Fig. 4.5 (a) TOE four-chamber view. (b) TOE 120° view. AoV, aortic valve.
(c) TOE 45° view. AoV, aortic valve. (d) TOE atrial septal view. (e) TOE transgastric
view. Mitral V, mitral valve.

Cardiac magnetic resonance imaging (cMRI)

Overview

Paediatric cMRI is usually undertaken in specialist cardiac centres. Patient movement degrades image quality so in some situations GA may be required. MRI does not involve ionizing radiation, and so is suitable for serial imaging.

cMRI is the gold standard imaging modality for the assessment of blood flow and cardiac function, including of the RV which may be difficult to image with TTE.

Clinical applications

- Tissue characterization and function in myocarditis, cardiomyopathy, and tumours.
- Prior to Fontan completion combined with CVP.
- Assessment of RV size and function in pulmonary hypertension.
- Qp:Qs assessment in shunt lesions.
- Post-tetralogy of Fallot repair assessment of pulmonary regurgitation and RV volumes.
- Aortopathy e.g. bicuspid aortic valve, Marfan syndrome.
- Additional uses include perfusion imaging and scar imaging.

> When combined with simultaneous invasive measurement of pressure via catheterization, the MRI-derived flow measurements can be used to accurately measure PVR and SVR. This requires extensive infrastructure and is not available in all cardiac centres (see p. 160).

Imaging the heart

- Most MRI scans are a composite image acquired over several heart beats.
- Cardiac and respiration motion can result in artefacts.
- Cardiac motion is accounted for with ECG gating.
- Respiratory motion can be overcome by:
  - Breath holding
  - Respiratory gating (tracking diaphragm motion and only acquiring at a certain position)
  - Averaging multiple images.

MRI sequences

- The typical MRI scan is comprised of multiple sequences to give a range of information that includes:
  - Visualization of blood vessels
  - Cine imaging of the heart including function
  - 3D assessment of the heart
  - Blood flow
  - Tissue characterization.
- Different sequences will be used, depending on the clinical indication for the scan.
- Sequence names vary from vendor to vendor, so the following descriptions are generic.

Black blood imaging
(See Fig. 4.6a.)
• Blood appears dark, useful for vessel wall imaging and assessment of stenosis.

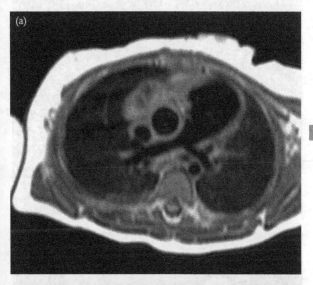

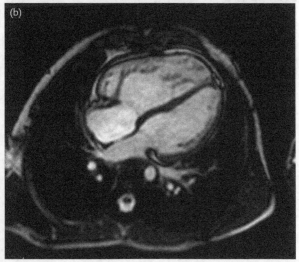

Fig 4.6 (*Contd.*)

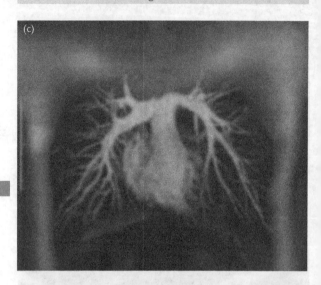

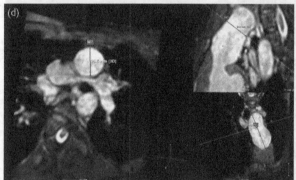

Fig. 4.6 (a) MRI black blood. (b) MRI cine four-chamber view. (c) MRI angiography. (d) MRI multiplane reformat of whole heart 3D volume showing neo-aorta in HLHS.

Cine imaging
(See Fig. 4.6b.)
- Multiple time points from several cardiac cycles acquired and brought together to create a moving image.
- Can be oriented to any plane.

Assessment of ventricular function
- Obtained from a short-axis stack of cine slices from the apex of the heart to beyond the inlet valves.
- Endocardial border is delineated at end diastole and end systole for each slice.
- These are summated to measure end-diastolic and end-systolic volumes.
- Stoke volume and ejection fraction are derived from these.

Phase contrast imaging
- Measures blood flow, including through whole cardiac cycle so useful for assessment of regurgitation.
- Also useful for shunt quantification (Qp:Qs).

MR angiography
(See Fig. 4.6c.)
- Injecting a gadolinium-based contrast agent and performing whole heart imaging to track the passage of the contrast through the circulation.
- Caution with use of MRI contrast where:
  - Established renal failure—risk of nephrogenic systemic fibrosis
  - Repeated administration risk of gadolinium deposition disease.
- Angiography not performed routinely.

Whole heart imaging (3D volume)
(See Fig. 4.6d.)
- High-resolution (1.0–1.5 mm) scan covering the entire heart.
- Useful for detailed evaluation of cardiac anatomy.
- Variety of post-processing tools available to maximize information.

Late gadolinium enhancement (scar imaging)
- Where there is disruption of cell membrane integrity, such as after an infarction, contrast distributes within the intracellular volume.
- The distribution of contrast allows for determination of the degree and location of an infarct or distribution of oedema within the myocardium.

Perfusion
- Perfusion imaging allows the passage of contrast through the heart to be visualized. Contrast will enter the coronary arteries creating higher-signal areas.
- Infusion of a potent vasodilator such as adenosine increases blood flow in healthy blood vessels. Fixed stenotic arteries will not be able to augment blood flow and so underperfused myocardial territories will show as darker areas.

Cardiac computed tomography (CT)

Overview

Like MRI, paediatric cardiac CT is usually undertaken in specialist centres. Unlike MRI, CT utilizes X-rays to image cardiac anatomy.

Recent developments such as dual source and multidetector arrays permit sub-millimetre spatial imaging and whole heart acquisitions in a single heartbeat, meaning that often GA is not required. It is important to consider the radiation dose, but modern technology has reduced this significantly.

Indications

Excellent special resolution, so is useful for:

- Angiography, especially coronaries
- Complex intracardiac anatomy and morphology
- Extracardiac anatomy and airway imaging.

Practicalities of acquisition

- Typically, an intravenous (IV) contrast dose is administered.
- A contrast bolus tracking sequence tracks the progress of contrast through the circulation.
- When maximal contrast is seen in the region of interest, the image volume is acquired.
- A breath hold will minimize respiratory motion (<10 sec).
- ECG-gated sequences are typically acquired in mid diastole.
- Contraindications: contrast reaction/allergy, clinical instability, renal impairment.

Image interpretation

Images can be viewed as a multiplane reformat, reconstructed into long-axis views, or displayed in 3D (Fig. 4.7).

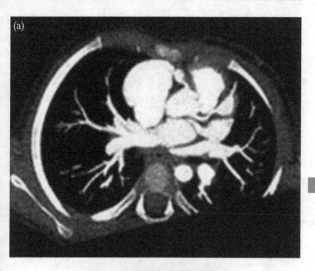

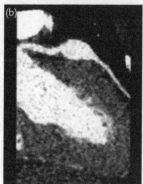

Fig 4.7 (Contd.)

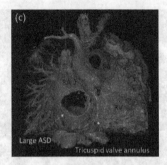

Fig. 4.7 (a) Axial CT with coronary aneurysms. (b) CT long-axis multiplane reformat reconstruction of the left anterior descending artery showing a medium-sized fusiform aneurysm. (c) CT 3D reconstruction of a heart demonstrating a large secundum ASD.

Cardiac surgery

Preoperative management

The preoperative review and decision-making process includes paediatric cardiologists, surgeons, anaesthetists, and intensivists. These discussions are formalized as a MDT meeting.

Advanced planning is essential for patients who require homograft material or a synthetic conduit or valve, so these can be ordered.

Preparing the patient

- Focused history and examination (including recent illnesses).
- Investigations:
  - Bloods: full blood count (FBC), urea and electrolytes (U&E), liver function tests (LFTs), clotting screen, cross-match (order packed red blood cells as per unit policy for neonate, infant, or child).
  - ECG.
  - CXR.
  - TTE.
  - Additional tests may be required where there are important co-morbidities.
- Consent including rationale for treatment, risks of mortality/and important morbidity.
- Patient should be nil by mouth (NBM) as per unit protocol.
- Check requirement for regular medications on day of surgery.
- Patients with cyanotic CHD and those who are arterial shunt-dependent, should be kept well hydrated while NBM to avoid acute increase in haematocrit. Local policies will determine whether this is with oral or intravenous fluids.
- Consideration should be given to stopping anticoagulants such as warfarin and aspirin when planning the procedure. Bridging heparin may be required, and local policies should be referred to.

Risk

Various risk scores are available, commonly used for research and audit purposes. Given the heterogeneous nature of CHD, it is important that a senior clinician discusses the individualized risk of each operation with the patient and/or family as part of the informed consent process.

Anaesthesia in children with cardiac conditions

Assessment for cardiac surgery or catheter intervention

The anaesthetist forms part of the MDT, making decisions about a patient's candidacy for intervention in all cases. In addition to the investigations outlined in the relevant chapters, anaesthetists will be interested in the following:

- Clinical condition: time may have elapsed since MDT decisions. In infants, feeding and growth and in older children, tiredness and self-limitation of physical activity may point to progression and need for up-to-date investigations.
- Intercurrent illnesses: all illnesses are considered in the context of the cardiac intervention and its urgency. Respiratory viral illnesses are the commonest issue and ideally children should be symptom free for at least 2 weeks prior to surgery (although this needs to be balanced with the risk of delaying urgent intervention).
- Comorbidities: respiratory, renal, and neurological conditions will all affect the risk profile of interventions (especially cardiopulmonary bypass (CPB)). All conditions should be optimized with the help of specialist teams where appropriate.
- Anaesthetic history: a detailed history should be sought of previous procedures including vascular access issues, airway management issues, and adverse reactions to medication.

Assessment and risk stratification for non-cardiac surgery and imaging

Children with CHD often have comorbidities that require non-cardiac surgical intervention. In addition, procedures may be required for vascular access, for feeding support, or imaging (CT, MRI, bronchoscopy, and diagnostic catheterization).

For such procedures the overriding consideration is often the risk of anaesthesia, as the intrinsic risk of the procedure is often low.

The general considerations of the anaesthetist are:
- *Indication for and intrinsic risk of the procedure*: this must be placed in the context of the intrinsic risk of anaesthesia for that child. Difficult cases should be discussed in an MDT setting.
- Patient's current clinical condition: especially where unstable or deteriorating
- Context of intervention within plans for cardiac condition: is the planned non-cardiac surgery needed prior to cardiac intervention, or might it best be delayed until after?

Risk stratification

Several systems have been published. The below summarises some common themes.

General considerations pointing to higher risk of anaesthesia are:
- Neonates and infants
- Ventricular dysfunction
- Inherited arrhythmia syndromes (LQTS, Brugada syndrome)
- Williams syndrome (especially with supravalvar AS)

- Recent cardiac surgery (<1 month).
- Inpatients—especially those requiring intensive support (ventilation, inotropes, renal replacement therapy).

High-risk cardiac lesions include:
- HLHS—prior to stage 1 or between stage 1 and 2 palliation
- Uncorrected cyanotic CHD
- Arterial shunt-dependent lesions and single ventricle physiology
- Severe LVOTO
- Pulmonary hypertension.

Moderate-risk cardiac lesions include:
- HLHS after stage 2 or 3 palliation (Glenn/Fontan circulation)
- Tetralogy of Fallot (presurgical correction)
- Complex but balanced cyanotic lesions (e.g. DORV, isomerism)
- Any lesion treated with PA bands
- Simple but symptomatic unrepaired intracardiac shunts: ASD, VSD, AVSD
- Repaired lesions with residual defects of haemodynamic significance.

Low-risk cardiac lesions include:
- Simple and asymptomatic intracardiac shunts: ASD, VSD
- PDA
- Fully repaired lesions (even initially complex ones) with minimal residual lesions

Planning of non-cardiac surgery

Planning should include:
- Understanding and consent for risks of anaesthesia as well as surgery
- Optimization of comorbidities
- MDT planning
- Planning of postoperative care—PICU/HDU where appropriate.

High-risk cases

High-risk lesions should be managed only in specialist centres with full cardiothoracic services. Anaesthetic care will usually be managed by the congenital cardiothoracic anaesthetic team. Contemporaneous cardiac assessment and investigation will be required and, except for minor surgery, often at least HDU care after.

Moderate-risk cases

Moderate-risk patients are in many ways the hardest to plan. Many will be manageable outside a specialist centre, especially for minor surgery, but this should be planned in close consultation with the cardiology and congenital anaesthesia team. Usually, cardiology review and imaging should have occurred with 3 months of anaesthesia.

In some cases (especially major surgery) and where they are at the more complex end of this spectrum, the team will make the decision to manage them in the cardiac centre, where the team can be supported by on-site congenital cardiac anaesthetic expertise and intensive care.

Low-risk cases

Low-risk lesions can be managed in non-specialist centres. Advice should be sought from the patient's primary cardiologist and any queries directed to the anaesthesia team. Usually, the imaging and information from annual review is sufficient unless the clinical condition has changed.

Cardiopulmonary bypass (CPB)

CPB involves the use of an extracorporeal circuit to temporarily take over the function of the heart and lungs during surgery. The aim is to provide a still, bloodless heart for surgery while the rest of the body remains perfused.

The circuit

The essential functions are circulation, oxygenation, ventilation, and temperature regulation.

1. Desaturated blood drains, by gravity, from the RA or venae cavae via venous cannulas to a reservoir.
2. A pump then propels blood through a membrane oxygenator (artificial lung) and an arterial filter.
3. Blood returns to the aorta via the aortic cannula.
   - Before instituting CPB the tubing is 'primed' with fluid and the patient is fully heparinized.
   - Protamine is given once CPB has been discontinued to reverse the action of heparin.

Physiological changes

During CPB there are changes in temperature, acid–base balance, non-pulsatile flow, circulating volume, and haematocrit. Additionally, the systemic inflammatory response is activated (thought to be due to the passage of blood though the non-endothelialized circuitry) and contributes to postprocedural end-organ dysfunction.

- Plasma protein system activation leads to a thrombogenic state.
- Platelets, neutrophils, monocytes, and lymphocytes are activated—the sequestration of neutrophils in the pulmonary vasculature increases capillary permeability leading to pulmonary oedema.
- Bleeding times do not return to normal until 4–12 hours after bypass.
- Increased capillary permeability leads to interstitial fluid shifts.
- Cortisol rises and remains high for 24 hours after bypass.
- Lung compliance and functional residual volume are reduced.
- Low perfusion pressure, haemodilution, and catecholamines impair renal function.

Myocardial protection

The heart is stopped with cardioplegia solution into the aortic root. High-potassium solutions are used to induce rapid diastolic arrest and minimize the depletion of high-energy phosphates.

Cerebral protection in aortic arch repairs

- *Deep hypothermic circulatory arrest*: the patient is cooled to a point (18–24 degrees Celsius) where bypass can be discontinued.
- *Antegrade (selective) cerebral perfusion*: the right common carotid artery via the brachiocephalic trunk or left common carotid artery are selectively cannulated with the aortic cannula. This allows perfusion of the brain at a lower bypass flow during surgery that requires opening the aortic arch. The organs below the descending aorta have no flow so are protected by moderate hypothermia (24-28 degrees Celsius).

Materials

Patches and baffles

Autologous pericardium

- *Pros*: widely available, sterile, non-antigenic, haemostatic.
- *Cons*: may thicken, fibrose, contract, or dilate. Glutaraldehyde fixation strengthens it helping with the ease of handling as well as reducing the risk of aneurysmal dilatation but at the cost of increased risk of calcification.

Cryopreserved homograft arterial wall

- *Pros*: haemostatic, conforms to contours.
- *Cons*: expensive, requires time to thaw, may stretch/dilate, calcify.

Dacron® (polyethylene terephthalate)

- *Pros*: strong, easily available, stable.
- *Cons*: stimulates inflammatory reaction causing adjacent fibrosis. Inelastic; not suitable for complex baffles in small spaces.

Gore-Tex®/Impra™ (expanded polytetrafluoroethylene (ePTFE))

Microporous synthetic polymer, derived from PTFE.

- *Pros*: conforms better than Dacron®, thus advantageous for baffles, less fibrous reaction than Dacron®.
- *Cons*: like Dacron® may be problems with needle-hole bleeding when used in high-pressure settings. Pores allow ingrowth of pseudo-intima.

Valves

Autografts

The use of one of the patient's own valves (e.g. pulmonary valve) moved to aortic position in the Ross procedure. Tissue will grow but may dilate.

Homografts

Donor human valves. Aortic and pulmonary roots are available; rarely used in aortic position due to calcification but much greater longevity in the pulmonary position.

Valved conduits

- Hancock valve: porcine valve within Dacron® tube—glutaraldehyde fixed.
- Contegra® valve: bovine jugular vein—glutaraldehyde-fixed bovine jugular vein with valve.

Bioprosthetic valves and mechanical valves

- Less commonly used in children.
- Mechanical valves require anticoagulation and serial replacement may be required to accommodate growth.

Surgery for shunt lesions: Atrial septal defect repair

Indication

Significant left-to-right shunt indicated by right heart volume loading.

Alternatives: selected secundum ASDs can be closed by a catheter-based device, and some superior sinus venosus defects may be treated via a covered stent which both closes the ASD and redirects the PVs.

Technique

The approach to repair is determined by the type of ASD. 'Primum' ASD (partial AVSD) repair is covered under repair of AVSD (see p. 132).

Secundum ASD

- Median sternotomy or lateral thoracotomy.
- Repair is with a patch closure technique via a right atriotomy, on bypass.
- If the defect is small, it can be directly sutured with continuous sutures.

Superior sinus venosus ASD

- The anatomy of the right PVs must be determined by careful mobilization of these structures.
- Care must be taken not to injure the sinoatrial node.
- The defect is patched to redirect the PVs to the LA.

If a PV drains high into the SVC the *Warden procedure* may be used: the SVC is transected just distal to the highest PV, and proximally oversewn. Through a RA incision, the ASD is closed with a patch, redirecting PV flow to the LA. The distal SVC is anastomosed to the RA appendage, restoring normal systemic venous return.

Risk

- 30-day mortality <1%.

Timing

- Usually between 2 and 5 years of age.

Specific complications

- Late pericardial effusions are common (15%).
- ASD predisposes to development of atrial arrhythmias, whether operated on or not. Atrial flutter and re-entrant tachycardias may occur around the patch or atriotomy scar.

Surgery for shunt lesions: Ventricular septal defect repair

Indication

Significant left-to-right shunt indicated by left heart volume loading. The aim is prevention of long-term complications of VSDs including pulmonary vascular disease, progressive ventricular dilation, and aortic insufficiency.

Technique

- Median sternotomy.

Perimembranous VSD

- Repair is via RA, through the tricuspid valve.
- The septal leaflet of the tricuspid valve may need to be retracted or detached.
- A patch (see p. 129) is used to close the defect.
- Care is taken to avoid the conduction tissue located at the inferior rim of the defect.

Muscular VSD

- Inlet and trabecular muscular approached as per perimembranous.
- The conduction bundle in inlet VSDs usually (not always) lies along the superior margin of the defect.
- Apical VSDs may need to be approached through a right ventriculotomy.
- Outlet VSDs may be approached through the MPA, RV if not accessible thorough the RA.
- VSDs below the moderator band may be difficult to locate/identify.
- A single patch may be used to close multiple defects if they are close together.

Doubly committed subarterial defects

- Repair through a pulmonary arteriotomy.
- The conduction axis is remote from the margins.

Risk

- 30-day mortality <1% (although up to 8% in 'Swiss cheese' defects or with other anomalies).

Timing

- Usually between 3 and 6 months, beyond 6 months this risk of pulmonary vascular disease increases.

Specific complications

- Residual VSD in 0.5% (missed defects, incomplete closure, reopening).
- Conduction disturbance: RBBB common, complete heart block 1%.

Surgery for shunt lesions: Atrioventricular septal defect repair

Indication
All AVSDs will require surgical repair.

Technique
- Median sternotomy.
- A single- or double-patch technique is used to repair the ventricular component followed by the atrial component.
- The size and shape of the patch is key in restoring competence to both AV valves.
- The zone of apposition between the bridging leaflets (confusingly sometimes also called the 'cleft') may be closed routinely to create a 'two-leaflet' valve or, depending on surgical preference, may be left open unless regurgitant.

Risk
- 30-day mortality 1–10% depending on anatomy, AV valve regurgitation, and associated lesions.

Timing
Complete AVSDs are usually repaired at around 6 months of age to avoid the development of pulmonary vascular disease and earlier, with higher risk, if major AV valve regurgitation. Partial AVSDs are usually repaired in early childhood.

Important considerations
Unbalanced AVSDs may be managed by single-ventricle palliation rather than septation to biventricular repair. Cases with 'borderline' size of LV are most difficult as it may not be possible to close the 'cleft'.

Specific complications
- Significant AV valve regurgitation in 10–15%, reoperation in 10%.
- Right bundle branch block (RBBB) 20%, complete AV block in 1%.
- Progressive left ventricular outflow tract obstruction

Surgery for shunt lesions: Pulmonary artery banding

Indication

Aims to limit pulmonary blood flow by reducing the luminal diameter of the MPA. This approach is used for many different lesions (often with excessive pulmonary blood flow) to 'buy time' until more definitive surgery is undertaken. Examples include multiple VSDs, coarctation of the aorta with a large VSD, late presentation of TGA, double-inlet LV without PS, ccTGA with tricuspid regurgitation.

Technique

- Median sternotomy (or left thoracotomy if concomitant coarctation repair).
- A band is placed around the PA and tightened to achieve distal PA pressure <50% of systemic pressure.
- Trusler and Mustard calculated optimal length of the band using the patient's weight in biventricular hearts (20 mm + weight (kg)).

Risk

- 30-day mortality <5% although can be higher in higher risk lesions

Timing

- Variable, depending on indication.

Important considerations

Removal of the band may be surgical (median sternotomy), or interventional by balloon dilation if additional surgical repair (VSD closure, arterial switch) is not required.

Specific complications

- PA distortion or stenosis
- Band migration

Surgery for left heart obstruction: Coarctation of the aorta repair

Indication

All neonatal 'duct-dependent' coarctation requires surgical repair. Some cases that present later in childhood can be managed with catheter-based intervention.

Technique

- Discrete coarctation of the aorta is usually approached via a left thoracotomy and repaired without bypass by end-to-end anastomosis (although other techniques are sometimes used).
- Coarctation with associated defects (e.g. VSD) or arch hypoplasia/ interruption is approached through a median sternotomy using CPB, with arch reconstruction as needed.

Management of associated VSD

A small concomitant VSD may be left untouched in anticipation of spon-taneous closure. Large VSDs may be closed as part of the same procedure or PA band applied and closure deferred if difficult surgical visualization/ access to defects.

Risk

- 30-day mortality <5%.

Timing

- Repair is usually shortly after presentation, allowing a period for recovery if possible end-organ damage.

Complications

Intraoperative
Spinal cord injury: reduce risk by short clamp time, avoiding acidosis, and measuring distal aortic pressure after clamping.

Early
- Rebound hypertension.
- Paraplegia.
- Renal failure in sick infants.
- Abdominal symptoms from mesenteric arteritis including pain, ileus, and, rarely, necrotizing enterocolitis (risk reduced if hypertension controlled).
- Chylothorax.
- Recurrent laryngeal nerve injury.

Late
- Re-coarctation in 10–45% of patients due to technically inadequate repair, hypoplasia of the arch proximal to the repair, or anastomotic stricture.
- Balloon dilatation may be indicated in younger children or stenting in older/larger children and adolescents

Surgery for left heart obstruction: Ross procedure

Indication

Performed for aortic valve disease (most commonly congenital AS). By using the patient's native pulmonary valve as an autograft, the problems of using a prosthetic aortic valve (need for anticoagulation, lack of growth) are avoided.

Technique

- Median sternotomy.
- Diseased aortic valve is excised, and coronary buttons are prepared.
- The pulmonary valve is excised, and anastomosed to the LVOT, with reimplantation of the coronary buttons.
- A pulmonary homograft is then used to restore continuity between the RVOT and PA.

Risk

- 30-day mortality <5%.

Timing

- Can be performed in neonatal life, but outcomes are better when performed later (late childhood)

Important considerations

It is essential to ensure that the pulmonary valve is normal (and so suitable to act as an aortic homograft).

Specific complications

- The pulmonary autograft will eventually fail (this can last 15–20 years in some cases), and this can happen early.
- The pulmonary homograft will also need to be replaced, again the timing is variable.

Surgery for cyanotic heart disease: Tetralogy of Fallot repair

Indication
All cases of tetralogy of Fallot will require surgical repair.

Technique
- Median sternotomy.
- VSD closure through the RA and relief of RVOTO which is often multilevel; may be subvalvar or supravalvar.
- Pulmonary valve and RVOT are accessed through the MPA.
- If the pulmonary valve annulus is too small, the PA incision is taken across the annulus and into the RVOT. It is then patched over with autologous pericardium, bovine pericardium, Gore-Tex®, or a 'monocusp' patch (transannular patch).

Risk
- 30-day mortality is 1–2%.

Timing
Complete repair is usually undertaken at around 6 kg/6 months of age but may be considered earlier if adequate branch PA size. Neonates with inadequate pulmonary blood flow due to severe RVOTO may undergo staged repair, with the first intervention to increase pulmonary blood flow with a ductal stent, a RVOT stent/patch, or a BTT shunt.

Important considerations
- Coronary arrangement: left anterior descending artery may arise from the right coronary artery and cross the RVOT.
- Branch PA size: hypoplasia may mean shunt/RVOT stent necessary prior to full repair to encourage growth.
- Tetralogy of Fallot with pulmonary atresia: adequate pulmonary vascular bed essential for repair so shunt/RVOT patch may be required. MAPCAs may need to be unifocalized to construct adequate vascular bed.
- Tetralogy of Fallot with absent pulmonary valve: PAs dilated, associated bronchomalacia ± compression by PAs leading to respiratory difficulty.

Specific complications
Early
- Arrhythmia, especially junctional ectopic tachycardia.
- Restrictive RV physiology.
- RV dysfunction (residual VSDs are poorly tolerated).
- Branch pulmonary artery stenosis

Late
- Residual/recurrent RVOTO.
- Pulmonary regurgitation with associated RV dilatation and dysfunction.
- Arrhythmias.
- Aortic dilation.

Surgery for cyanotic heart disease: Arterial switch operation

Indication

Operation of choice for neonates with TGA/intact ventricular septum, and (when combined with VSD repair) TGA with VSD and DORV with subpulmonary VSD.

Technique

- Median sternotomy.
- Single-stage anatomical correction: transection of aorta and PA, PA anastomosis to aortic root and anastomosis of the ascending aorta to the PA root.
- Both coronary arteries are 'harvested' as 'buttons' (a rim of aortic wall around the ostia) from the aorta and reimplanted into the neo-aortic root (originally the PA).
- *Lecompte manoeuvre*: used to bring the MPA anterior to the aorta. Avoids the need for an interposition graft to connect the neo-pulmonary root to the PA bifurcation, by bringing it anterior to the ascending aorta.

Risk

- 30-day mortality for the most common coronary arrangements is 2%.

Timing

Neonates may require initial intervention with balloon atrial septostomy. Surgical repair is usually performed electively within the 2 weeks of life. Patients with a large VSD may be repaired later.

Important considerations

- Coronary artery anatomy is highly variable and important to define: some variations of coronary anatomy confer an increased risk, in particular intramural coronary arteries.
- There are some contraindications to arterial switch: LVOTO (unless resectable), severe abnormalities of the pulmonary valve (this will become the systemic 'neo-aortic valve'), and late presentation with an involuted LV.

Specific complications

Early
- Coronary artery malposition/kinking leading to coronary ischaemia.
- Branch PA narrowing after the Lecompte manoeuvre.
- PA/aortic stenosis at the anastomosis.

Late
- Aortic root dilatation ± aortic valve regurgitation.

Surgery for cyanotic heart disease: Nikaidoh procedure

Indications

TGA with PS or pulmonary annular hypoplasia.

Technique

- Median sternotomy.
- The aortic root (lying anteriorly) is excised from the RVOT with a skirt of muscle.
- The coronary arteries either detached and reimplanted once aorta is moved or moved en bloc with the aorta.
- The pulmonary valve (lying posteriorly) is excised and the septum between the aortic and pulmonary root is divided.
- The aortic root is translocated into the space thus created over the LVOT.
- The VSD is closed with a patch or using the skirt of muscle on the translocated aorta.
- The Lecompte manoeuvre is performed bringing the PA anterior to the aorta.
- RV to PA continuity is restored with a conduit or patch.

Surgery for cyanotic heart disease: Rastelli procedure

Indication

TGA with VSD and PS or specific variants of DORV.

Technique

- Median sternotomy.
- The LV is connected to the aortic valve using a baffle (patch of Dacron/Gore-Tex®), through the VSD.
- Easiest when the VSD is a large perimembranous VSD.
- The RV connected to the PA with a valved conduit (homograft, bovine jugular vein, or Hancock valved conduit).

Specific complications

- The RV–PA conduit will need to be changed when the child outgrows it, or earlier if there is conduit stenosis.
- Sub-AS may develop if the VSD becomes restrictive.

Surgery for cyanotic heart disease: Mustard/Senning procedure (atrial switch)

Indication

These were widely employed in the past for treatment of TGA. Their application has largely been superseded by use of the arterial switch operation.

Technique

- Median sternotomy.
- *Mustard operation*: the atrial septum is excised, and a large patch of autologous pericardium is used to form an intra-atrial baffle, directing systemic venous flow to the mitral valve and the pulmonary venous flow to the tricuspid valve.
- *Senning operation*: redirection is by cutting and folding of the native atrial tissues, usually without the use of extraneous material.

Risk

- 30-day mortality is <5% for both these procedures.

Specific complications and outcomes

- *Mustard*: constriction of the venous pathways, baffle leaks, sinus node dysfunction, atrial arrhythmias.
- *Senning*: systemic venous pathway obstruction.

With either approach the RV remains the systemic ventricle with risk of late RV failure.

The 20-year survival is 80–90% for both these operations. VSD at time of surgery is a risk factor for late reoperations.

Surgery for Functionally Single Ventricle disease: Norwood procedure

Indication

Most commonly performed for HLHS and other conditions characterized by severe left heart hypoplasia. It is the first procedure in the three-stage surgical approach culminating in total cavopulmonary connection (Fontan circulation)

The aim is to secure unrestricted systemic and pulmonary venous return to the heart with the cardiac output being balanced between the pulmonary and systemic vascular beds.

Technique

- Median sternotomy.
- Atrial septectomy to ensure unobstructed pulmonary venous return which bypasses the LV.
- Fashioning of a DKS anastomosis with repair of the aortic coarctation and augmentation of the aortic arch:
  - MPA is transected proximal to the bifurcation and distal PA closed.
  - The arterial duct is transected, and ductal tissue is excised.
  - The aortic coarctation is excised and continuity between the aortic isthmus and descending aorta is ensured.
  - The diminutive ascending aorta is anastomosed to the transected proximal MPA (DKS anastomosis) and a patch is used in augmentation of the aorta from the DKS to the descending aorta.
- Provision of controlled pulmonary blood flow: either a systemic-to-PA shunt—3–4 mm PTFE graft between the innominate artery and the right PA (BTT shunt), or RV–PA conduit—usually a 5 mm Gore-Tex® tube, from the RV to the left (Sano shunt) or right (modified Sano shunt) PA.

Risk

Procedural mortality 5–30%. Substantial interstage (between stage I and II) mortality of 5–15%. Home monitoring (of oxygen sats/weight) and close review until stage II has been shown to reduce risk.

Risk factors for poor outcome include weight <2.5 kg, restrictive atrial communication at presentation, small ascending aorta, tricuspid regurgitation, late presentation, prematurity, and mitral stenosis with aortic atresia.

Timing

- Usually performed within the first week of life.

Important considerations

RV–PA conduits (Sano modification) may confer a more stable immediate postoperative course due to the reduction in diastolic runoff from the systemic to pulmonary circulation seen with a BTT shunt. However, the ventriculotomy required for a Sano shunt ventricle raises concern for the function of the RV in the long term.

Aspirin is used to maintain shunt patency. Additional antiplatelet therapy or systemic anti-coagulation may be required, particularly where the is concern about shunt integrity.

Specific complications

Early
- Arrhythmia.
- Arch obstruction.
- Shunt occlusion.
- Imbalance of Qp:Qs.

Late
- Atrial restriction.
- Obstruction at DKS level.
- Shunt occlusion.
- Progressive tricuspid valve regurgitation
- Poor ventricular function.
- The best reported outcomes are of an 80% survival to completion of the Fontan circulation

Surgery for Functionally Single Ventricle disease: Superior cavopulmonary connection

This includes the Glenn shunt and hemi-Fontan procedure.

Indication

Intermediate procedure in the three-stage palliation of conditions in which the LV is not adequate to support the systemic circulation (i.e. between Norwood and Fontan). Also used in situations in which the RV is not able to support the pulmonary circulation. Results in all deoxygenated blood from upper body passing directly into the pulmonary circulation via the SVC

Technique

* Median sternotomy.

Glenn shunt

* Usually performed on a beating heart without the need for cardioplegic cardiac arrest.
* The inferior end of the SVC is anastomosed to the upper border of the right PA.

Hemi-Fontan

* The SVC is not transected at the RA junction, but an opening made in the posterior wall of the SVC, extending onto the RA junction.
* This opening is then anastomosed to a corresponding opening in the RPA.
* The anastomosis is separated from the RA by a patch.
* Cardioplegia and arrest of the heart is necessary due to the intracardiac component of the procedure needed for patch closure of the SVC–RA junction.
* Facilitates lateral tunnel method of completion Fontan.

Risk

* 30-day mortality <5%.

Timing

* Usually electively between 3 and 6 months of age.

Important considerations

* Assessment of growth of branch PAs prior to the procedure (e.g. with CT).

Specific complications

Early

* 'SVC syndrome'—swollen head/face if PVR high.
* Thrombosis.
* Obstruction of SVC to PA anastomosis (more commonly with Glenn)
* Sinus node dysfunction

Late

* Development of aortopulmonary collaterals.

Surgery for Functionally Single Ventricle disease: Fontan completion (total cavopulmonary connection)

Indication

This is the final element of the staged approach to single-ventricle palliation. Usually performed >1 year after Glenn/hemi-Fontan operation. Requires low PA pressure and low PVR, as bloods returns passively from the systemic circuit (without a subpulmonary ventricle).

Technique

- Median sternotomy.
- The IVC flow is directed to the pulmonary circulation. This separates the systemic and pulmonary circulations so that they are in series. Two main variants:
  - *Intracardiac total cavopulmonary connection (lateral tunnel)*: performed with cardioplegic arrest and occasionally with circulatory arrest.
  - *Extracardiac total cavopulmonary connection* using a conduit to take blood from the IVC to PAs. Can be performed on the warm beating heart.
- In both cases, aim for early extubation to improve Fontan haemodynamics (positive pressure ventilation reduces systemic venous return/filling).
- A fenestration may be created between the systemic venous circulation and the RA to allow deoxygenated blood to shunt into the systemic circulation (thus acting as a 'pop-off' valve to maintain cardiac output should PVR rise). The role of fenestration is controversial and practice varies between cardiac surgical centres

Risk

- 30-day mortality <5%.

Timing

- Usually electively between 3 and 5 years of age.

Important considerations

Selected patients should be in in sinus rhythm, have adequately sized PAs, and good ventricular function. The absence of any one of these increases the risk of poor outcome.

Specific complications

Early

- Prolonged chest drainage not uncommon and often the cause for delay in discharge. Effusions are usually serous, occasionally chylous. If >2 weeks, assessment of the anatomy and haemodynamics with cardiac catheterization ± CT/MRI should be considered.
- Potential interventions include enlargement/creation of fenestration or balloon/stent to branch PAs.

Late
- Risk of thromboembolism requires lifelong "anti-platelet therapy e.g. aspirin or anticoagulation e.g. warfarin" (see p. 284).
- Atrial arrhythmias.
- Development of collateral vessels (leading to large left-to-right shunts and contributing to volume loading of the ventricle).
- Ventricular failure.
- Fontan associated liver disease (FALD)
- Plastic bronchitis
- Protein-losing enteropathy (see pp. 152–154).

Extracorporeal membrane oxygenation (ECMO)

- Also known as extracorporeal life support (ECLS).
- Can be used in children >2.5 kg.

The ECMO circuit

Oxygenator (silicone membrane oxygenator, hollow fibre oxygenator), pump (centrifugal or roller pump), heat exchanger, bubble detectors, in-line blood gas and saturation monitors, and flow measurement device.

Indication

- Acute, severe, reversible cardiac or respiratory failure where oxygenation and/or cardiac output cannot maintain life despite optimal conventional treatment.
- In the context of cardiac surgery, ECMO may be used immediately postoperatively to support cardiac output/cardiac function until spontaneous recovery of function or to allow time for further investigation to treat underlying cause of circulatory compromise.
- Common respiratory indications include:
  - Congenital diaphragmatic hernia
  - Meconium aspiration syndrome
  - Primary pulmonary hypertension of the newborn
  - Respiratory distress syndrome.

Types

Venovenous
Usually for pure respiratory failure. VV ECMO does not provide cardiac support to assist the systemic circulation. In infants <10 kg this is via a double-lumen cannula in the internal jugular vein. In children >10 kg there may be two separate cannulas draining from a femoral vein and reinfusing into the jugular vein.

Venoarterial
Usually for cardiac failure or respiratory failure where there is cardiac compromise. Most cannulation is through the jugular vein and common carotid artery by cut down in the neck. Venting of the left heart may be achieved through an ASD, or a vent placed through the right superior PV or left atrial appendage.

Complications

- *Mechanical*: clots or air in circuit, oxygenator failure, and pump failure.
- *Cannula*: mediastinal bleeding, carotid artery, and aortic dissection.
- *Neurological*: thromboembolic, intracranial bleeds, and seizures.
- *Other*: pneumothorax, tamponade, cardiac ischaemia, overwhelming sepsis, coagulopathy, infection, renal failure, gastrointestinal haemorrhage, and ischaemia.

Outcomes

Current survival rate after ECMO for neonatal respiratory failure is 77%, and paediatric respiratory failure 56%. Extracorporeal cardiopulmonary resuscitation is the use of ECMO to salvage patients with cardiorespiratory arrest. For this indication, in children survival to hospital discharge is 40%.

The single-ventricle circulation

The Fontan circulation

Background

When considering the approach to repair of any form of CHD, a fundamental consideration is 'can the heart be repaired to a normal biventricular circulation or not?'.

Where biventricular repair is not feasible, a 'functionally single-ventricle circulation' will be considered. This is usually because of one of the following reasons:

- The left heart is not sufficiently developed to support the systemic circulation (e.g. HLHS).
- The right heart is not sufficiently developed to support the pulmonary circulation (e.g. tricuspid atresia).
- More complex intracardiac anatomy (e.g. straddling AV valves sometimes precludes biventricular repair).

The Fontan repair leaves the SVC(s) and IVC draining directly to the pulmonary circulation (see p. 148). Blood flow to the lungs is maintained by passive systemic venous pressure rather than by active contraction of a subpulmonary ventricle. This leads to chronically elevated systemic venous pressure and reduced cardiac output which is a major contributor to late complications and Fontan failure.

The surgical approach is usually staged (i.e. Norwood operation, (see p. 142), superior cavopulmonary connection (e.g. Glenn operation) (see p. 144), and Fontan operation (see p. 146)).

Good function of the dominant systemic ventricle, minimal AV valve regurgitation, good respiratory function, low PVR, and absence of obstruction in any part of the circulation are essential for an optimally functioning single-ventricle circulation.

Imaging of the single-ventricle circulation

- Echocardiography is the modality of choice to confirm the diagnosis in advance of initial surgery.
- CT or MRI is helpful where vascular anatomy is complex (CT may also provide more detailed information about the lungs, e.g. pulmonary lymphangiectasia, and MRI provides functional data but is more likely to require GA).
- *Pre-Glenn imaging*: CT, MRI, or cardiac catheterization to delineate the systemic venous anatomy and the PAs. Echocardiography to assess AV valve regurgitation and echocardiography/MRI for ventricular function.
- *Pre-Fontan imaging*: echocardiography and MRI to assess vascular anatomy, ventricular function, and AV valve regurgitation. Cardiac catheterization to measure PA pressures/estimate PVR or for intervention prior to Fontan completion. In some centres measurement of a central venous pressure is undertaken at the time of MRI in lieu of cardiac catheterization.

Outpatient approach to the single-ventricle patient

- Height, weight, BP, pulse oximetry, and 12-lead ECG at each visit.
- Holter monitoring at intervals depending on symptoms.
- Echocardiography to assess ventricular function, AV valve regurgitation, and systemic and pulmonary pathways.

- Detailed imaging (CT/MRI or catheter) prior to surgical procedures. During later follow-up, CPET to objectively assess effort tolerance and MRI to assess cardiac function and Fontan pathways, as echo visualization becomes more difficult.
- Screening for liver dysfunction undertaken from teenage years at latest (e.g. by liver ultrasound scan with elastography, with MRI if concerns).
- In addition to cardiac investigations attention should also be paid to:
  - feeding and nutrition
  - recognition and impact of comorbidities
  - psychological, developmental and educational support

Medications commonly used in single-ventricle patients

- See Chapter 15 for more details.
- Aspirin or anticoagulation (warfarin) because of risk of thrombosis, choice dependent on surgical approach and unit preference.
- ACEi used selectively for cardiac function or AV valve regurgitation.
- Diuretics perioperatively or long term in selected patients.
- Antiarrhythmics as appropriate.

Precautions/recommendations in single-ventricle patients

- Physical activity should be encouraged to enhance muscle pump augmentation of venous return.
- Infective endocarditis prophylaxis varies by country and institution.
- GA should only be undertaken by an anaesthetist who is confident and experienced with single-ventricle physiology and where PICU care is available.
- Positive pressure ventilation may impede venous return.

Outcomes and the failing Fontan

Long-term considerations

- The long-term prognosis after completion of a functionally single-ventricle circulation is guarded.
- Exercise tolerance is reduced due to the absence of a subpulmonary ventricle.
- Progressive deterioration of ventricular function also occurs due to the underlying substrate combined with abnormal loading conditions and myocardial ischaemia.
- AV valve regurgitation may worsen with time.
- Arrhythmias are frequent and antiarrhythmic drugs or pacemaker implantation may be required.
- Specific complications include protein-losing enteropathy, hepatic fibrosis/cirrhosis, and plastic bronchitis.
- Increased risk of stroke and other thrombotic complications (hence most units use low-dose aspirin or anticoagulation, e.g. warfarin).
- Heart transplantation may be an option for some patients but may be precluded either by the patient's condition or donor availability.

The failing Fontan circulation

- This may manifest itself in a number of ways including:
  - Functional deterioration
  - Exercise intolerance
  - Failure of growth
  - Shortness of breath
  - Increasing level of cyanosis
  - Ascites
  - Peripheral oedema
  - Coagulopathy.
  - Development of organ-specific complications such as plastic bronchitis (protein-losing enteropathy).
- Symptoms develop late in the progression of disease so careful surveillance is essential.
- Late failure is largely a reflection of chronic venous congestion coupled with reduced cardiac output.
- Modifiable factors are investigated and treated, including:
  - *Arrhythmias*: chronotropic incompetence, atrial arrhythmias
  - *Fontan pathway obstruction*: exclusion by CT/MRI/catheter
  - *Optimization of ventricular function*: medical therapy, e.g. diuretics, afterload reduction
  - *Optimization of cardiac mechanics*: e.g. conversion of atriopulmonary Fontan to extracardiac technique, surgical repair of AV valves.
- Organ-specific complications need investigation and therapy:
  - *Plastic bronchitis*: characterized by shortness of breath and expectoration of rubbery 'casts' of the bronchial tree. Treated with steroids, inhaled mucolytics, pulmonary vasodilators, azithromycin, lymphatic investigation, and occlusion in selected cases.
  - *Protein-losing enteropathy*: characterized by protein loss into the gut, with subsequent low serum protein and oedema. Treated with steroids (oral budesonide), heparin, enlargement of Fontan

fenestration, and occlusion of abnormal gut lymphatics in selected cases.
• *Liver fibrosis/cirrhosis*: screening from around 10 years after Fontan, with blood tests and ultrasound with elastography, with MRI if concerns. Management is supportive. Combined heart/liver transplantation has been performed.

Cardiac catheterization and intervention

Introduction

Cardiac catheterization is performed in children for diagnostic and/or interventional purposes. The aim of diagnostic catheterization is to obtain haemodynamic information, such as BP or blood flow, in order to inform future management decisions. Compared to previous eras, diagnostic catheterization is less commonly performed, as information about complex anatomy and blood flow is increasingly gained from MRI and CT rather than invasive angiography.

Cardiac catheterization involves the insertion of a catheter into the heart itself as well as the great arteries and veins, most commonly via the femoral artery or vein. The catheter is manipulated within the heart and great vessels to measure pressures. During the procedure it is also possible to:

- Sample blood to measure PO_2, PCO_2, acid–base status, and oxygen saturations.
- Inject radiopaque contrast medium to image the anatomy.
- Perform intravascular ultrasound (e.g. for post-heart transplant assessment of coronary arterial narrowing).
- Perform cardiac interventions.

ECG and arterial pressure monitoring take place throughout the procedure, which in children is performed under GA. Most cardiac catheterization procedures are performed as day-case or single overnight stay procedures.

Preparing the patient

- Focused history and examination (including recent illnesses).
- Investigations: this is institution dependent, but may include bloods (FBC, U&E, LFTs, clotting screen), ECG, CXR, and TTE.
- A group and save may be sufficient for diagnostic catheterization and non-aortic arch interventions. In children <10 kg in weight and for aortic arch interventions, blood is usually cross-matched (also institution dependent).
- Informed consent.
- Patient should be NBM, and consideration should be given to whether any of their regular medication should be withheld.
- Patients with cyanotic CHD and those who are shunt dependent, should be kept well hydrated while NBM to avoid acute increase in haematocrit. Local policies will determine whether this is with oral or intravenous fluids
- Consideration should be given to stopping medications that affect the clotting cascade when planning the procedure.

Post-procedure checks

- Lower limb pulses, BP, vascular access puncture site (for bruising or swelling).
- CXR, TTE (procedure dependent).

Common complications

The rate of serious complications following most cardiac catheter procedures is low, with a mortality of <1%. Risk factors include the following:

- *Patient-related factors*: younger age, smaller size, anticoagulant medication use, bleeding disorders, polycythaemia, connective tissue disorders, multiple previous cardiac surgeries or repeated catheterizations using the same vascular access site.
- *Procedural factors*: use of larger sheaths in small patients, complex procedures, unplanned access site, simultaneous ipsilateral venous and arterial femoral access impacting tissue perfusion.

The management of intraprocedural complications is outside the scope of this handbook, but some specific complications that may be identified by the ward team caring for the patient are listed below:

Bleeding from vascular access site

Apply firm pressure over the bleeding site and request review if persists.

Contrast reaction

This is usually mild but should be documented. Signs include generalized warmth and flushing. More severe reactions include urticaria and laryngeal oedema. Senior help should be sought if reaction suspected and treatment with antihistamine ± corticosteroids considered.

Loss of lower limb peripheral pulses

May be due to thrombus or arterial spasm. A poorly perfused, cold limb needs urgent senior review. Pulses may also be checked with a Doppler probe. Consideration of heparinization or treatment to dissolve clots (e.g. tissue plasminogen activator) should be considered according to institutional policy.

Hypotensive, tachycardic patient

Consider:
1. Hypovolaemia due to occult blood loss (e.g. retroperitoneal haemorrhage)
2. Pericardial effusion — investigate with urgent TTE (see p. 316).

Infection

If post-catheterization pyrexia persists, bloods including cultures should be taken before giving antibiotics.

Haemodynamic assessments

The following measurements are usually taken as part of a full haemo-dynamic assessment during diagnostic catheterization (for normal values see Table 7.1):

- Oxygen saturations: IVC; SVC; innominate vein; RA; RV; PA.
- Right heart pressures: RA ('a' wave, 'v' wave, mean); RV (systolic, end-diastolic); PA (systolic, diastolic, mean); pulmonary capillary wedge pressure (PCWP) ('a' wave, 'v' wave, mean).
- Left heart pressures: LA (systolic, diastolic, mean); aorta (systolic, diastolic, mean); LV (systolic, end-diastolic).

Some useful calculations

Using the data collected as outlined above, the following calculations can be used: (such calculation cans also be useful in the operating theatre (see box 7.1)).

Shunt calculation by oximetry (Qp:Qs)

1. Measure SVC oxygen saturation ('sats'), IVC sats, and pulmonary vein sats.
2. Calculate *mixed venous sats = $(3 \times SVC\ sats + IVC\ sats)/4$*.
3. Then calculate *Qp:Qs = (aortic sats − mixed venous sats)/(pulmonary vein sats − PA sats)*.

Cardiac output (CO) using Fick equation

1. Calculate *arterial O_2 content = arterial sats $\times$ 1.36 $\times$ Hb*.
2. Calculate *mixed venous O_2 content = mixed venous sats $\times$ 1.36 $\times$ Hb*.
3. Calculate *arteriovenous oxygen difference ($AVDO_2$) = arterial − mixed venous oxygen content*.
4. Estimate O_2 consumption (VO_2)—either from nomograms (may be inaccurate) or directly measured (technically difficult).
5. Calculate *CO = $VO_2/AVDO_2$*
6. Calculate *cardiac index (CI) = CO/BSA*.

Pulmonary vascular resistance (PVR)

1. Calculate *transpulmonary gradient (TPG) = mean pulmonary artery pressure (mPAP) − (mean left atrial pressure (mLAP) or mean pulmonary capillary wedge pressure (mPCWP) or left ventricular end diastolic pressure (LVEDP))*.

Table 7.1 Normal values

Site	Pressure (mmHg)	Oxygen saturation (%)
RA	3–5 (mean)	65–80
RV	22–26 / 3–5 (systole / end-diastole)	65–80
PA	12–26 / 8–12 (systole / diastole) 10–20 (mean)	65–80
PCWP	5–8 (mean)	—
LV	85–125 / 4–7 (systole / end-diastole)	98–100
Aorta	85–125 / 40–80 (systole / diastole)	98–100

2. Calculate $PVR = TPG/CO$ (gives result in mmHg/L/min or Wood units).
3. Calculate indexed PVR ($PVRI$) = TPG/CI (normal <3 Wood units.m²). (Multiply × 80 to convert to dynes.sec.cm⁻⁵.m².)

Notes on cath lab calculations

- VO_2 is rarely measured directly (requires mass spectroscopy) and instead is assumed to be between 130 and 180 mL/min/m² in infants and children/young adults, respectively (these estimates represent a significant potential source of error).
- Supplemental oxygen and hyperoxia affects VO_2, dissolved oxygen, and haemodynamic calculations using the Fick equation.
- In the absence of a cardiac shunt, *thermodilution* is an alternative method of assessing pulmonary blood flow/cardiac output.
- The gold standard method for assessment of flow is MRI and in specialized centres combined MRI and catheterization allows for the simultaneous measurement of invasive pressures and MRI-derived flow to accurately measure PVR.
- Haemodynamic calculations can also be useful in the operating theatre (see box 7.1).

Acute vasodilator testing

- In patients with CHD with shunt lesions, vasoreactivity testing can be performed to evaluate the possibility of repair, measuring the variability of PVR in different conditions.
- It is also used in pulmonary arterial hypertension (PAH) to identify patients who may be candidates for treatment with pulmonary vasodilators
- Usually performed by calculating PVR with administration of both high inspired oxygen (FiO₂ 0.8–1.0) and inhaled nitric oxide (20 ppm), following measurement of PVR during an initial baseline condition.

Box 7.1 Rapid assessment of Qp:Qs in the operating theatre

Following surgical closure of some lesions (e.g. VSD), there may be doubt about the haemodynamic significance of any residual shunts. In this setting, a 'saturation run' may be undertaken by the surgeon to assess the significance of the residual shunt:

$$Qp:Qs = \frac{\text{Systemic arterial sats} - \text{mixed venous sats}}{\text{PV sats} - \text{PA sats}}$$

- Systemic arterial sats: sats of arterial blood gas or pulse oximetry saturation.
- Mixed venous sats: surgical sampling of RA blood.
- PV sats: typically assumed to be 100% or LA sat measured.
- PA sats: directly measured by surgeon from PA.

Atrial septal defect closure

Transcatheter closure with a device is the first choice for secundum ASD closure when morphology is suitable. Several devices by different manufacturers are available.

Procedure

- TOE imaging most commonly used; TTE or intracardiac imaging may suffice.
- Femoral venous access is most common; alternatively, internal jugular vein or transhepatic approach.
- Systemic heparinization and antibiotic coverage as per institutional protocols.
- A diagnostic catheter study may be performed if indicated.
- The atrial septum is crossed with the catheter ± wire.
- The size of the defect is measured (various techniques can be used), to allow selection of an appropriate device.
- The device is passed to the LA through a delivery sheath.
- The device is then deployed, with one disc on the LA side of the septum and the other on the RA side using imaging guidance.
- A stability check can be performed by pushing and pulling the device.
- The device is detached from the delivery cable and released.

Post-procedure

- Post-procedural TTE and ECG prior to discharge, focusing on device position, competence of AV valves, and absence of pericardial effusion.
- Minimum of 6 months of aspirin therapy. In some units dual antiplatelets or a longer period of therapy is preferred.

Follow-up

- Follow-up policy varies by institution but should include an early check of device position and to exclude complications and lifelong follow-up as per manufacturer's recommendation.
- Perforation of the heart or adjacent structures by the device (cardiac erosion) is rare. It occurs most commonly in the first 24–48 hours after implantation, but also may occur years later.

Patent ductus arteriosus occlusion

Transcatheter occlusion of PDA is now the first-choice procedure for all age groups outside of the neonatal period and is also commonly performed in premature neonates (with a device CE marked for infants weighing as little as 700 g). TTE is usually sufficient to select cases for occlusion, but CT is sometimes used to define the anatomy of the duct in complex cases. Several devices including duct-specific devices and coils are available.

Procedure

- Pre-procedurally if high PVR is suspected (e.g. in the setting of bidirectional PDA flow), right heart haemodynamics evaluation is mandatory.
- Femoral venous ± arterial approach is preferred. Femoral artery access only may be sufficient when the PDA is small and using a coil is anticipated. Femoral venous access only is appropriate for neonatal duct occlusion.
- Systemic heparinization and antibiotic coverage as per institutional protocols.
- The lateral projection is the main projection to measure the size and shape of the PDA prior to deployment.
- After deployment, an angiographic catheter is positioned at the level of the ductal ampulla in the aorta and angiography is performed to demonstrate the position of PDA occluder.

Post-procedure

- Post-procedure TTE before discharge, focusing on residual shunt and exclusion of complications, including impingement on left PA flow by the device.
- No post-procedure medications are required.

Follow-up

- Follow-up timings vary according to institutional policy but will include an early check of device position and to exclude complications including partial obstruction of the origin of the LPA or descending aorta by protrusion of the device.
- It may be appropriate to discharge from follow-up as early as 1 year after procedure if no residual cardiac lesions.

Balloon pulmonary valvuloplasty

Transcatheter ('balloon') pulmonary valvuloplasty is the first-line treatment for isolated valvar PS. It can be performed in all age groups including neonates and adults.

Procedure

- Femoral venous access is most common; alternatively, internal jugular vein or transhepatic approach.
- Systemic heparinization and antibiotic coverage as per institutional protocols.
- A diagnostic catheter study to assess RV pressures and pulmonary valve gradient should be performed.
- RV angiography allows assessment of the size of the pulmonary valve annulus.
- An appropriate guidewire is manipulated to a distal branch PA (or descending aorta if the arterial duct is patent) and a low-pressure balloon ~90–150% size of the annulus is selected.
- Reassessment of pressure should be performed aiming to achieve a systolic RV pressure <50% of the arterial pressure and a pulmonary valve gradient <20 mmHg.

Post-procedure

- Post-procedural TTE prior to discharge, focusing on pulmonary valve Doppler gradient and excluding complications.
- No post-procedural medications are required.

Follow-up

- Dependent on age at time of procedure: neonates should be followed up within a few weeks, older patients can be seen ~8–12 weeks post-procedure.
- Lifelong follow-up but if PS and pulmonary regurgitation remain no more than mild, unlikely to require future interventions.

Percutaneous pulmonary valve implantation

Transcatheter pulmonary valve implantation is considered to be the first-line treatment for patients with severe pulmonary valve stenosis/regurgitation and adequately sized vessels for vascular access. It can be performed in patients with native pulmonary valve dysfunction or in surgically implanted conduits or bioprostheses. Preprocedural imaging by CT/MRI is mandatory to assess whether the RVOT dimensions are suitable for pulmonary valve implantation.

Procedure

- Femoral venous access is most common; alternatively, internal jugular vein or transhepatic approach.
- Systemic heparinization and antibiotic coverage as per institutional protocols.
- A diagnostic catheter study to assess RV pressures and pulmonary valve gradient should be performed.
- RV angiography and sizing balloon interrogation allows assessment of the size and compliance of the RVOT/conduit. Simultaneous coronary angiography allows assessment of the proximity of the coronary arteries.
- An appropriate guidewire is manipulated to a distal branch PA and a delivery sheath advanced to the MPA.
- An appropriately sized transcatheter valve is chosen and deployed in the RVOT with or without pre-stenting.

Post-procedure

- TTE prior to discharge, focusing on pulmonary valve Doppler gradient and excluding complications.
- CXR imaging to assess stented valve position and orientation as a baseline for future surveillance.
- Post-procedural antiplatelet agent as per institutional protocol (although there is evidence that lifelong aspirin prolongs valve longevity).

Specific complications

- RVOT/conduit rupture (can be treated by covered stent implantation).
- Coronary artery compression by stented valve—rare if appropriate periprocedural assessment undertaken.
- Early/late endocarditis—more common if PS indication, some valves may be more prone to infection than others.

Follow-up

- Outpatient review ~8–12 weeks post-procedure with TTE ± CXR.
- Surveillance of ventricular volumes and function as per institutional protocols.
- Lifelong follow-up and repeat procedures will be required; current valve longevity estimated to be ~8–12 years.

Balloon aortic valvuloplasty

Transcatheter ('balloon') aortic valvuloplasty can be performed as a treatment for AS in all age groups from neonates to adults. Procedural results and freedom from reintervention are similar to surgical aortic valve repair.

Procedure

- Femoral arterial access is most common; alternatively, common carotid or axillary artery access may be used.
- Systemic heparinization and antibiotic coverage as per institutional protocols.
- A diagnostic catheter study to assess LV pressures and aortic valve gradient should be performed.
- Ascending aortic angiography allows assessment of the aortic valve annulus and coronary artery anatomy.
- An appropriate guidewire is manipulated across the aortic valve to the LV and a suitable balloon ~80% of the annulus size is chosen.
- Post-valvuloplasty assessment of LV pressure and aortic valve gradient should be undertaken. TTE or TOE assessment of the degree of aortic regurgitation may be useful if considering increasing balloon size.

Post-procedure

- TTE prior to discharge, focusing on aortic valve Doppler gradient and severity of regurgitation and excluding complications.
- No changes to regular medication are usually required.

Specific complications

- Ventricular arrhythmias during the procedure may occur, a defibrillator should be available in the catheter laboratory.
- Aortic regurgitation is common, if less than moderate it is usually well tolerated. If severe and associated with symptoms, early aortic valve replacement may be required.

Follow-up

- Dependent on age at time of procedure; neonates should be followed up within a few weeks, older patients can be seen ~8–12 weeks post-procedure.
- Patients will require lifelong follow-up but if AS and aortic regurgitation remain no more than mild, they are unlikely to require future interventions.
- Surveillance for associated aortopathy is appropriate for all patients with congenital AS.

Electrophysiology studies in children

Radiofrequency catheter ablation is a safe and effective treatment for a wide range of arrhythmias. Depending on the type of arrhythmia, there is an ~90% long-term success rate. Complication rates are around 1–2% (including vascular damage, cardiac tamponade, and AV nodal injury). Most arrhythmias are medically managed until the child is at least 15–20 kg in weight to avoid the higher complication rates seen in smaller children.

Procedure details

- The procedure is generally carried out under GA in children, but older children and teenagers can tolerate even long procedures with appropriate local analgesia and sedation.
- The majority of cases are carried out using femoral venous access (usually both sides), but left-sided ventricular tachycardias, or more complex arrhythmias in CHD, may necessitate arterial or alternative venous (i.e. internal jugular) access.
- It is increasingly common in children to use 3D mapping systems to position catheters and guide ablation (requiring little or no fluoroscopy).
- Several diagnostic catheters are placed in standard positions to carry out the diagnostic electrophysiology study: typically, in high RA, bundle of His, coronary sinus, and RV.
- Pacing manoeuvres and medication (commonly isoprenaline and adenosine) are used to assess both baseline characteristics and then to induce and define the clinical tachycardia.
- When the arrhythmia substrate and location has been identified (e.g. an accessory pathway in atrioventricular re-entry tachycardia (AVRT)), an ablation catheter is used to cause an endocardial scar and block conduction of the arrhythmia, either using radiofrequency or cryoablation energy.

Balloon atrial septostomy

Creates/enlarges an atrial communication to facilitate interatrial mixing of blood (e.g. patient with TGA or complex single-ventricle anatomy.

Procedure

- Femoral venous or umbilical vein access (neonates) are most common.
- Systemic heparinization and antibiotic coverage as per institutional protocols.
- Can be performed under TTE guidance at the bedside or in the catheter laboratory using fluoroscopy.
- A balloon atrial septostomy catheter is manipulated from the IVC to the RA and across the atrial septum to the LA. The balloon is inflated and withdrawn to the RA rapidly to create a tear in the atrial septum.

Post-procedure

- TTE focusing on the atrial septum and excluding complications.
- No changes to regular medication are usually required (although in some patients the improved mixing at atrial level may allow the prostaglandin infusion to be reduced or stopped).

Specific complications

- Damage to intracardiac structures may occur when the balloon is inflated and withdrawn. Careful monitoring with TTE during the procedure may help avoid this.
- Cerebral emboli are relatively common, although these may not be clinically apparent.

Follow-up

- Ongoing inpatient surgical planning is usually required depending on anatomy.

Pericardiocentesis

Accumulation of pericardial fluid may result in impairment of ventricular filling and cardiac tamponade. Percutaneous pericardiocentesis can be undertaken either in an emergency situation, or as an elective procedure with a more chronic accumulation.

Procedure

- Can be performed at the bedside on the intensive care unit or in the cardiac catheter laboratory. Conscious sedation is usually required, and GA should be given cautiously due to the risk of haemodynamic upset in the presence of cardiac tamponade.
- If GA is used, the cardiologist should prepare all necessary pericardiocentesis equipment in advance in case of haemodynamic deterioration on induction of anaesthesia.
- Echocardiographic guidance is helpful and the subxiphoid approach is usually preferred to minimize the risk of damage to surrounding structures.
- The fluid can be aspirated via a needle or sheath and an in-dwelling catheter (drain) may be left *in situ* in case of early re-accumulation.
- Samples should be sent for biochemical analysis, microscopy, and histology.

Post-procedure

- Total drainage volume (procedural and post-procedural) should be measured and recorded.
- The drain should be removed when no longer required. If there is persistent drainage (>48 hours) then steroid therapy may be helpful to reduce the degree of pericardial inflammation.

Specific complications

- Damage to cardiac structures, pleura, or liver may occur when the needle is passed to the pericardial space.

Genetics and paediatric cardiology

Introduction

- The majority of CHD is non-syndromic, and secondary to multifactorial, environmental, and polygenic causes. However, CHD may be associated with a range of genetic abnormalities ranging from chromosomal aneuploidy through to single-gene disorders. CHD can be isolated or associated with extracardiac manifestations.
- Around 30% of patients with CHD have syndromic phenotypes which can include developmental delay and/or extracardiac manifestations.
- Recognition of associated conditions is important for optimization of patient care.
- This chapter will focus on the most common genetic syndromes that are associated with CHD.

Patau syndrome (trisomy 13)

Incidence
• 1 per 20,000 live births.

Clinical features
• CHD:
  • Occurs in 80%.
  • Cardiac defects include VSD, ASD, AVSD, tetralogy of Fallot, and DORV.
• Holoprosencephaly.
• Omphalocele, anal atresia, and congenital diaphragmatic hernia.
• Characteristic features:
  • Cleft lip and/or palate.
  • Microphthalmia/anophthalmia.
  • Postaxial polydactyly.

Genetics
• The majority of cases are caused by primary trisomy 13 (an extra copy of chromosome 13 in every cell).
• A small proportion of cases are caused by an unbalanced translocation (often due to a parental Robertsonian 13;14 translocation).
• A few cases will be secondary to mosaic trisomy 13 (an extra copy of chromosome 13 in a proportion of cells).

Prognosis
• Around 50% of liveborn infants will die within the first week of life.
• Less than 10% will survive beyond 1 year of life.
• These longer-surviving individuals often have mosaic trisomy 13.

Edward syndrome (trisomy 18)

Incidence
- 1 in 10,000 live births.

Clinical features
- CHD:
  - Occurs in around 90% of individuals with trisomy 18.
  - Most common cardiac defects are perimembranous VSD, often with malalignment of the aorta and valve dysplasia.
- Characteristic features:
  - Microcephaly, ventriculomegaly.
  - Oesophageal atresia, diaphragmatic hernia.
  - Kidney abnormalities, hypospadias.
  - Micrognathia.
  - Unilateral club hand (radial aplasia).
  - Low-set ears.
  - Clenched or overlapping fingers.
  - Rocker bottom feet.

Genetics
- The majority of individuals have primary trisomy 18 (an extra copy of chromosome 18 in every cell).
- Around 6% have mosaic trisomy 18 (an extra copy of chromosome 18 in a proportion of cells) or partial trisomy 18 (part of chromosome 18 is duplicated in all cells) This may be a result of a balanced translocation in one of the parents.

Prognosis
- Around 50% of live-born infants will die within the first week of life.
- Less than 5% will survive beyond 1 year of life. These individuals often have mosaic trisomy 18.

Down syndrome (trisomy 21)

Incidence

- 1 in 1000 livebirths (this is ~50% less than expected due to screening and subsequent termination of pregnancy).

Clinical features

- CHD:
  - Seen in 40–50% of individuals with trisomy 21.
  - The most common cardiac defects are AVSD, VSD, tetralogy of Fallot, PDA, and ASD.
- Gastrointestinal anomalies: duodenal atresia/stenosis, Hirschsprung's disease.
- Hypothyroidism.
- Developmental delay and learning difficulties.
- Characteristic features:
  - Flat facial profile.
  - Brachycephaly.
  - Up-slanting palpebral fissures.
  - Protruding tongue.
  - Widened sandal gap.
  - Single palmar crease.

Genetics

- The incidence of trisomy 21 increases with maternal age.
- 95% of cases are caused by non-disjunction, resulting in primary trisomy 21 (an extra copy of chromosome 21 in every cell).
- Around 2–3% of cases are caused by a Robertsonian translocation (usually 14;21), which is often familial.
- A further 2% of cases are caused by mosaicism (an extra copy of chromosome 21 in a proportion of cells) and 1% caused by a variety of chromosome rearrangements.

Follow-up

- All babies with trisomy 21 should have cardiac review with echocardiogram within 6 weeks of birth.
- Feeding, growth, potential upper airways obstruction, thyroid function, and hearing (glue ear) all require monitoring. Growth should be plotted on Down syndrome-specific growth charts.
- Affected babies with CHD are at risk for early pulmonary vascular disease. Watch for upper airways obstruction and occult aspiration.
- Improved results of cardiac surgery are improving longer-term survival. Early-onset dementia complicates later course.

Turner syndrome (45, X0)

Incidence
- 1 in 2000 female live births.

Clinical features
- CHD:
  - Usually left-sided, including coarctation of the aorta, bicuspid aortic valve, and hypoplastic left heart.
  - Also associated with aortic dilatation (see p. 184).
- Oedema: hydrops or increased nuchal translucency in pregnancy, and oedema of the hands and feet in the neonatal period which may persist.
- Short stature.
- Renal: horseshoe kidney and other structural anomalies.
- Primary amenorrhoea. Most are infertile.
- Characteristic features:
  - Webbed neck.
  - Wide-spaced nipples.
  - Cubitus valgus.
- Susceptibility to autoimmune disease.

Genetics
- The majority of fetuses with Turner syndrome will spontaneously miscarry in a pregnancy.
- Around 50% of females with Turner syndrome have a single X chromosome (45, X0).
- The remainder have structural rearrangements of the X chromosome or sex chromosome mosaicism.

Follow-up
- Monitoring of growth, secondary sex characteristics, osteoporosis, BP, thyroid function, and diabetes.
- Middle ear infections may cause hearing loss.
- May require growth hormone and/or sex hormone replacement therapy.
- Multidisciplinary review including cardiology, endocrinology, nephrology, gynaecology, ENT, and psychology.
- Individuals can survive into adulthood but there is a slightly reduced life expectancy in Turner syndrome due to acquired cardiovascular disease such as thoracic aortic aneurysm (dissection), hypertension, stroke, coronary artery anomalies, and acquired disease.

22q11 deletion syndrome

Incidence

- 1 in 4000 live births.

Clinical features

- CHD:
  - Most commonly outflow tract abnormalities such as tetralogy of Fallot, common arterial trunk, and interrupted aortic arch.
  - VSD, ASD, and PDA are also common.
- Cleft palate or velopharyngeal insufficiency.
- Hypocalcaemia (hypoparathyroidism).
- Immunodeficiency (reduced T-cell subsets).
- Kidney abnormalities.
- Arthritis.
- Developmental delay or learning difficulties.
- Behavioural or mental health problems including attention deficit hyperactivity disorder, autism, and schizophrenia.

Genetics

- 22q11 deletion syndrome is caused by a microdeletion on the long arm of chromosome 22.
- In 90% of cases these occur *de novo* but in 10% the deletion is inherited from a parent. The parent may have few symptoms.
- The condition is transmitted in an autosomal dominant pattern.

Follow-up

- Multidisciplinary review including cardiology, cleft, nephrology, ENT, infectious disease, audiology, feeding, and speech and language therapy.
- Early prognosis heavily impacted by cardiac lesion and degree of immune deficiency.
- Late psychological/psychiatric manifestations require prompt recognition and input.

Williams syndrome

Incidence

- 1 in 7500–10,000 live births.

Clinical features

- CHD:
  - Occurs in ~80% of individuals with Williams syndrome.
  - Typical cardiac defects are supravalvular AS and branch PA stenosis; 25% have supravalvular PS.
- Endocrine: hypercalcaemia, hypothyroidism.
- Overfriendly 'cocktail party' personality in younger children.
- Developmental delay and learning difficulties.
- Characteristic features: periorbital fullness, fullness of the cheeks and lips, wide mouth, bulbous nasal tip, widely spaced teeth, and stellate iris.
- Skeletal and joint problems (progressive): scoliosis, kyphosis.
- Chronic ear infections ± hearing loss.

Genetics

- Williams syndrome is caused by a chromosome deletion on the long arm of chromosome 7 (7q11.23), encompassing the elastin gene (*ELN*), the loss of which is thought to be responsible for the cardiac and connective tissue abnormalities associated with this condition.
- In the majority of affected individuals, this deletion occurs *de novo*.

Follow-up

- Clinical guidance for screening in William syndrome changes from infancy to adulthood.
- These include cardiovascular monitoring, growth and endocrine screening, coeliac screening, genitourinary assessment, and serum and urinary calcium studies.
- General anaethesia: this has elevated risk in the face of significant supravalvar AS due to coronary involvement. Cardiological advice should be sought.

Noonan syndrome

Incidence
* 1 in 1000–2500 live births.

Clinical features
* CHD:
  * Pulmonary valve stenosis.
  * Peripheral PA stenosis.
  * HCM.
  * Other cardiac lesions (e.g. VSD, tetralogy of Fallot, and ASD).
* Short stature.
* Lymphatic dysplasia (e.g. lymphoedema, chylothorax, and intestinal lymphangiectasia).
* Haematological abnormalities (abnormal clotting with easy bruising).
* Characteristic features:
  * Hypertelorism, ptosis.
  * Low-set and posteriorly rotated ears.
  * Short, webbed neck.

Genetics
* Noonan syndrome is a heterogeneous condition that has clinical overlap with other conditions (such as Costello or cardiofaciocutaneous syndrome) within the same cell signalling pathway.
* Collectively, these conditions are known as RASopathies.
* 40% of Noonan syndrome cases are caused by heterozygous pathogenic variants in *PTPN11*.
* The remainder are caused by variants in other RASopathy genes such as *SOS1*, *RIT1*, and *RAF1*.
* The condition is transmitted in an autosomal dominant pattern in ~50% of cases. In the remainder the pathogenic variant occurs *de novo*.

Follow-up
* Regular cardiac screening, haematological assessment, neurodevelopmental follow-up, and growth assessments in childhood.
* Children with a height at least 2.5 standard deviations below the mean or with low IGF-1 levels are eligible for growth hormone treatment.

CHARGE syndrome

Incidence

- 0.1–1.2 in 10,000 live births.

Clinical features

- CHARGE syndrome is a highly variable condition associated with multiple congenital anomalies as well as developmental delay.
- The most frequently associated features which make up the acronym are:
  - **C**oloboma: present in 80–90%, can affect the iris, retina, choroid, or discs.
  - **H**eart defects: occur in 70–85% of patients and are often complex. The most common conditions are tetralogy of Fallot, aortic arch abnormalities, and septal defect.
  - Choanal **A**tresia: this can be unilateral or bilateral and affects around half of patients with CHARGE.
  - Growth **R**etardation/**R**enal abnormalities.
  - **G**enital abnormalities.
  - **E**ar anomalies and sensorineural hearing loss. Dysplasia of semicircular canals in 99%.

Genetics

- CHARGE syndrome is caused by a heterozygous pathogenic variant in the gene *CHD7*.
- This change is usually *de novo* in the affected individual.

Follow-up

- As CHARGE syndrome can be clinically variable, every child with a suspected or confirmed diagnosis should have baseline cardiac, ophthalmological, ENT, urogenital, growth, and neurodevelopmental assessments. Most children with CHARGE are developmentally delayed.
- Psychological issues (e.g. autistic features or obsessive–compulsive traits) may emerge in later childhood. Musculoskeletal abnormalities (e.g. truncal hypotonia/scoliosis) later in childhood or adolescence.

Alagille syndrome

Incidence

- 1 in 30,000–70,000 live births.

Clinical features

- CHD:
  - Peripheral PA stenosis.
  - Tetralogy of Fallot.
  - Other CHD.
- Prolonged neonatal jaundice (caused by hypoplasia of intrahepatic bile ducts) causing liver disease.
- Butterfly vertebrae.
- Posterior embryotoxon on inner surface of cornea.
- Characteristic features:
  - Deep-set eyes.
  - Prominent chin and forehead.
  - Long nose.

Genetics

- Pathogenic variant of gene *JAG1* (>90%), or chromosome 20 deletion encompassing *JAG1* gene (7%), or heterozygous *NOTCH2* pathogenic variant (2%).
- In 30–50% of cases, the condition is inherited from an affected parent.
- Autosomal dominant inheritance.

Follow-up

- Patients should have regular liver function, cholesterol, triglycerides, bile acids, and clotting studies. Malabsorption can lead to deficiency of fat-soluble vitamins (A, D, E, K).
- A baseline cardiac and ophthalmic assessment as well as AP spinal X-ray and renal ultrasound should be carried out.
- Failure to thrive is common and expert dietary input and supplementation is often required.
- In 15% progressive liver disease results in cirrhosis with potential need for liver transplantation. Careful cardiac assessment is mandatory as part of assessment.

Holt–Oram syndrome

Incidence
- 1 in 100,000 live births.

Clinical features
- CHD:
  - Present in around 75% of patients.
  - Most commonly ASD or VSD.
  - More complex lesions are also seen.
- Cardiac conduction defects such as sinus bradycardia or heart block. Conduction problems can be progressive.
- Upper limb malformations: typically, triphalangeal or absent thumb, phocomelia, and radial anomalies.

Genetics
- Holt–Oram syndrome is caused by heterozygous pathogenic variants in a gene, *TBX5*.
- The condition is transmitted in an autosomal dominant pattern.

Follow-up
- Management of CHD and orthopaedic anomalies as appropriate.
- ECG should be carried out annually and pharmacological treatment may be required for arrhythmias.

VACTERL association

Incidence

- 1 in 10,000 – 40,000 live births.

Clinical features

- **V**ertebral defects.
- **A**nal atresia.
- **C**ardiac defects: these occur in 40–80% of affected individuals.
- **T**racheo-o**E**sophageal fistula.
- **R**enal anomalies / **R**etardation of growth
- **L**imb abnormalities.

Genetics

- The abnormalities that occur in this condition are seen more frequently than would occur by chance, hence they are grouped together as an 'association'.
- To date, no single unifying genetic cause has been identified.
- It is important to explore the differential diagnoses, such as CHARGE syndrome, 22q11 deletion syndrome, Fanconi syndrome, and others to allow appropriate management and accurate recurrence risk counselling.
- Intelligence is typically normal.

Management

- Management is dictated by the nature of the anomalies in any individual case.

Inherited aortopathy

Ascending aortic diseases (dilatations, aneurysms, dissections) are rare but important causes of morbidity and mortality in children and young adults. Prevalence in the paediatric age group is largely unknown but aortic dissections were found in approximately 5% of autopsies performed for sudden cardiac deaths in young individuals.

Atherosclerosis and other acquired cardiovascular stressors and risk factors which lead to aortic and vascular disease progression in adults are virtually absent in children. Defects in structural components of the connective tissue (i.e. collagen, elastic fibres), components of the smooth muscle cells contractile apparatus (ACTA2, MYH11), or abnormal signalling in the tumour growth factor (TGF)-β pathway can disrupt the arterial wall integrity and eventually cause aortic dilatation and lead to acute aortic events.

In *syndromic aortopathies*, the diagnosis is often clinical and based on the multiple associated features:

Marfan syndrome

- Key phenotypic features are in the cardiovascular, skeletal, and ocular system, diagnosis is based on Ghent nosology.
- Aortic root dilatation develops early and is present in up to 90% of individuals by the age of 19 years.
- Around 2% require aortic surgery in childhood.
- Median age at elective surgery or type A dissection at 32–36 years old.
- Surgical aortic diameter threshold >45–50 mm.
- Caused by heterozygous, pathogenic variants in Fibrillin 1(FBN1).
- 75% of cases it is inherited from an affected parent (autosomal dominant). 25% are *de novo*.

Loeys–Dietz syndrome

- Frequent cardiovascular, skeletal, and craniofacial defects.
- Presents with more aggressive and diffuse vascular pathology than Marfan syndrome starting with aortic root dilatation and spreading to other portions of the arterial tree.
- Aortic dissection rate approaching 70% of patients in early reports and for smaller diameters.
- Mean age at first vascular procedure is 20 years old.
- Surgical aortic diameter threshold >42 mm (echocardiography) or 44 mm (CT/MRI).

Non-syndromic heritable thoracic aortic disease

- Up to 20% of patients referred for repair of thoracic aneurysm or dissection have familial clustering of the disease in the absence of other phenotypic features.
- Inheritance is usually autosomal dominant.
- Dissection can occur at normal diameters with the most severe genotypes.
- Surgical aortic diameter threshold: no consensus recommendation.

Bicuspid aortic valve

- Bicuspid aortic valve (BAV) is the most common congenital heart defect (0.5-2%) and is often found in healthy asymptomatic individuals.
- Familial nature is recognized along with specific genetic mutations (e.g. NOTCH1, ROBO4).
- Bicuspid aortic valve aortopathy is progressive and impacted by associated aortic valve stenosis ± regurgitation.
- The ascending aorta rarely merits surgical intervention in children.
- Around 50% of young men with bicuspid aortic valve have abnormal aortic dimensions at root and/or ascending aortic level. Approximately 5% of patients will develop an aortic dissection.
- Risk of dissection for larger diameters compared to connective tissue diseases.

Turner syndrome

- In addition to the CHD mentioned in the section on Turner syndrome (see p. 176), aortic dilatation is reported in 45% and up to 5% experience dissection or rupture at relatively small diameters, often in the third or fourth decades of life.

Vascular (type IV) Ehlers–Danlos syndrome

- A connective tissue disorder, affecting blood vessels in all areas of the body but particularly medium- and large-diameter arteries including the aorta.
- Other features include translucent skin, easy bruising, and rupture of hollow organs such as the colon.
- Vascular EDS is caused by heterozygous pathogenic variants of the COL3A1 gene and is transmitted as an autosomal dominant trait but more than 50% are de novo.

Clinical management of aortopathy

- Diagnosis is based on accurate familial and personal family history, examination and clinical genetic review, echocardiogram, and/or cross-sectional imaging.
- Patients with inherited aortopathy and proven connective tissue disease are at substantially increased risk of acute aortic complications (dissection, rupture) with major mortality associated.
- Outcomes of elective surgery are superior to emergency repair and current international guidelines advocate a focus on risk stratification, regular monitoring with imaging, medical treatment (beta-blockers and angiotensin receptor blockers), and prophylactically replacing the diseased aortic segment once the diameter reaches a threshold based on the underlying condition.
- PEARS (personalised external aortic root support) procedure is becoming more common as a surgical strategy.

Genetic testing and congenital heart disease

- Referral or advice from clinical genetics colleagues can be helpful in the diagnosis of rare genetic conditions.
- There are several types of genetic tests available, and it is important to understand the differences between these. Conventional karyotype analysis and fluorescence *in situ* hybridization (FISH) are less frequently used in modern laboratory practice.

Chromosome tests

- *Quantitative fluorescence-polymerase chain reaction (QF-PCR)*: this technique is used to amplify specific regions of DNA and quantify the amount present in those regions. It is a rapid test that is useful in pregnancy or in the neonatal setting when urgent quantification of certain chromosomes (13, 18, 21, and sex chromosomes) is needed to guide management.
- *Microarray or comparative genomic hybridization (CGH) or SNP array*: a detailed chromosome test which looks for deletions and duplications in the chromosomes but would also detect a chromosome aneuploidy. Useful when a chromosomal diagnosis is suspected, such as Williams syndrome or 22q11 deletion syndrome. If there is a high suspicion of a trisomy but the QF-PCR is normal, the array test may detect chromosomal mosaicism. This test will not detect a balanced or Robertsonian translocation, or triploidy.

Monogenic conditions

- It is possible to test for monogenic conditions in numerous ways.
- If the condition is inherited and the familial pathogenic variant is known, analysis for the same variant in DNA from the affected relative can be requested.
- For aortopathies, cardiomyopathies and arrhythmias a panel of genes can be requested
- When the phenotype is not definitive and there are several differentials, a better approach would be to request a CHD panel or whole exome/ genome sequencing, depending on your institution's guidelines.
- In the NHS, the National Genomic Test Directory can guide clinicians on what genetic tests are available and the eligibility criteria (see https://www.england.nhs.uk/publication/national-genomic-test-dire ctories/).

Recurrence of CHD

- When a parent has CHD and an underling genetic cause has been identified, the recurrence risk for future pregnancies will be based on the inheritance pattern of that genetic condition (see OMIM: Online Mendelian Inheritance in Man; https://www.omim.org/).
- When CHD has been identified in a child with a genetic syndrome, inheritance studies can be arranged on parents to advise the future offspring risk (if a pathogenic variant has been identified in the child).
- In the majority of syndromic cases described in this chapter, the condition would have occurred for the first time in the child ('*de novo*'),

therefore future offspring risk would be low if neither parent was affected with the syndrome. However, there is always a small risk due to gonadal mosaicism in one of the parents.
- In cases of isolated CHD, the recurrence risk to future siblings is less straightforward and based on data from large cohorts of patients.
- The recurrence rate is typically 2–3% but depends on the cardiac lesion.

Fetal cardiology

Introduction

Virtually all major forms of CHD, as well as some minor forms, can be detected during fetal life with a high degree of diagnostic accuracy.

Prenatal diagnosis

- Allows parental choice and time to plan optimal perinatal care.
- Has been shown to improve survival rate after birth and improve long-term neurological outcome for some CHD lesions.

Confirming normality can provide reassurance to parents at high risk of having a child with CHD.

Fetal circulation and neonatal adaptation

The fetal circulation differs fundamentally from the postnatal circulation. This is critical to the understanding of normal adaptation to postnatal life and the impact of CHD.

- During fetal life, delivery of O_2 and nutrition to the fetus is via the placenta.
- Both the LV and RV supply the systemic arterial circulation in contrast to postnatal life (Fig. 9.1).
- Oxygenated blood returning from the placenta passes into the umbilical vein which connects to the heart via the ductus venosus where the blood accelerates and preferentially streams right to left across the foramen ovale.
- The LV faces the low-resistance cerebral and placental circulations.
- Less oxygenated blood enters the RV and is pumped into the PA where most blood is shunted through the arterial duct into the descending aorta.
- The lungs are fluid-filled with high PVR, so they receive far less blood than they do postnatally.
- There are near-equal atrial and ventricular pressures in the right and left sides of the heart, with low systemic arterial pressure due to the low-resistance placental circulation.
- Thus, the *fetal circulation is a low-pressure, high-volume parallel circulation.*
- At birth, the lungs inflate as the baby takes their first breaths leading to a marked fall in PVR and increase in pulmonary blood flow.
- Once the umbilical cord is clamped there is an increased SVR and rise in systemic arterial BP.
- Increased pulmonary venous return leads to an increase in LA pressure causing closure of the foramen ovale.

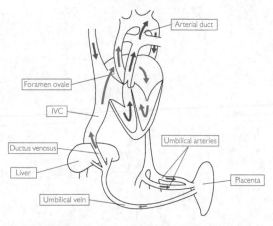

Fig. 9.1 Fetal circulation and transition to postnatal circulation.

- The fall in PVR and rise in SVR leads to left-to-right shunting at ductal level.
- Constriction/closure of the arterial duct occurs in response to increased oxygenation and other endothelial mediators.
- Taken together, these changes result in separate pulmonary and systemic arterial circulations which work in series postnatally.
- Cardiovascular changes are summarized in Table 9.1.

Table 9.1 Cardiovascular changes during the transition from fetal to postnatal circulation

	Prenatal	Transitional (first days)	Postnatal
Ventricular pressures	LV = RV	LV > RV	LV >> RV
Atrial pressures	RA ~ LA	RA ~ LA	LA > RA
Foramen ovale	Open, R → L	Open, L → R or closed	Closed
Arterial duct	Open, R → L	Open, L → R	Closed
PVR	High	Reducing	Low
SVR	Low	High	High

L, left; R, right.

The circulatory changes assume normal cardiac structure and represent the usual pattern of postnatal adaptation. Understanding this normal physiology explains the pattern of presentation of CHD:

- Most CHD will not cause cardiac failure during fetal life because of patency of shunts; e.g. in HLHS the RV supports the systemic circulation via the arterial duct.
- Lesions such as significant VSD, AVSD, and PDA present with clinical signs of heart failure when PVR has fallen as this allows for significant left-to-right shunt and resultant pulmonary over-circulation.
- In contrast, lesions with duct-dependent systemic or pulmonary blood flow present as the arterial duct constricts.

Antenatal screening for congenital heart disease

- The majority of CHD occurs in a low-risk population and can only be detected by population screening using obstetric ultrasound.
- High-risk groups are usually additionally referred for detailed fetal echocardiography. Referrals may be from general practitioners (GPs), midwives, or obstetricians and are made to tertiary centres for detailed evaluation of the heart.

Screening low-risk groups to detect CHD

- Currently, five views of the fetal heart are included in the fetal anomaly scan protocol to aid detection of CHD:
  1. Abdominal situs view.
  2. Four-chamber view.
  3. View of aorta from LV.
  4. View of PA from RV.
  5. Three-vessel tracheal view.
- The success of prenatal screening is related to the expertise and experience of the sonographers performing the scans, and regional differences in detection rates remain.

Timing of scans

- Fetal anomaly scans are generally performed at 18–22 weeks of gestation.
- Some specialist fetal cardiology centres can perform fetal cardiology scans from 13–14 weeks of gestation.
- The majority of fetal cardiac scans are performed between 18 and 23 weeks of gestation.

High-risk groups for CHD

These groups may be referred for fetal echocardiography, in addition to standard population screening. See Table 9.2.

Maternal risk factors

- Family history of CHD in a first-degree relative (of the fetus): the risk to the next generation is between 1.5% and 3%.
- Maternal diabetes: risk of cardiac malformation 2–3% (good diabetic control in early pregnancy is thought to diminish the risk).
- Exposure to teratogens in early pregnancy: risk of cardiac malformation 2–3%, depending on exposure.

Table 9.2 Recurrence risk of CHD

Previous children affected with CHD	Recurrence risk
One	2–3%
Two	10%
Three	~50%

Fetal risk factors

- The detection of some extracardiac fetal anomalies on ultrasound can be associated with CHD and should lead to a complete examination of the fetal heart.
- Abnormalities in more than one system should arouse the suspicion of an underlying genetic condition.
- Fetal arrhythmias: may be associated with structural heart disease, particularly complete heart block.
- Non-immune fetal hydrops may be due to CHD or arrhythmia.
- Increased nuchal translucency in the first trimester is associated with a high risk for CHD, even when the fetal karyotype is normal.

What can and what cannot be detected

The differences between the fetal and postnatal circulation mean some defects will only become evident after birth.

- Not all forms of cardiac malformations are detectable prenatally.
- Parents should be made aware of such limitations.

Abnormalities that can be detected

- Major cardiac structural abnormalities.
- Moderate to severe obstructive lesions of aorta and PA:
  - Moderate to severe AS/PS.
  - Coarctation of the aorta.
- Abnormalities of cardiac function.
- Rhythm disturbances:
  - SVT, atrial flutter, VT.
  - Congenital heart block.
  - Irregular rhythm.

Abnormalities that cannot be or may not be detected

- Secundum ASD.
- Persistent arterial duct.
- Mild forms of obstructive lesions of aorta and PA.
- Some forms of VSD.

Management and counselling

Following prenatal diagnosis of CHD, the parents are provided with detailed information including the following:
- An accurate description of the anomaly.
- Information regarding the need for surgical or catheter intervention:
  - The type of treatments available for the condition.
  - The number of procedures likely to be required.
  - The associated mortality and morbidity.
  - The long-term outlook for the child through to adult life.
- A major decision for the parents is whether they wish to continue with the pregnancy or not.
- There is a high association with other anomalies, so further investigations by a fetal medicine team should be offered to exclude any associated lesions.
- The finding of an associated anomaly may influence the parents' decision about how to proceed.
- In continuing pregnancies, multidisciplinary perinatal management can be planned:
  - The parents can meet the paediatricians, paediatric cardiologists, and paediatric cardiac surgeons likely to be looking after their baby.
  - Prenatal diagnosis will allow planning for immediate cardiac assessment of the neonate and avoid late diagnosis after an infant has become cyanotic or acidotic.
  - In some cases, the site of delivery can be changed for delivery to take place in a unit with paediatric cardiology facilities on site (see p. 198).
- In selected cases, some parents may feel unable to opt for termination of pregnancy, but in view of the poor prognosis for their baby may opt for 'comfort care' after birth:
  - The baby is kept comfortable using medical management, but no active surgical management is undertaken.
  - The baby is allowed to die of their CHD.
  - Involvement of the neonatal and palliative care teams is vital, and this can happen before birth.

Considerations for delivery of the fetus with congenital heart disease

Considerations for delivery of the fetus with congenital heart disease

Once the diagnosis of CHD is made, and the parents choose to continue with the pregnancy, appropriate planning for delivery and perinatal management of the fetus is vital for effective care.

Site of delivery

- Options include a specialist obstetric unit with cardiology input, or local obstetric unit, with advantages and disadvantages to each option.
- The nature of the CHD is extremely important as well as the perceived need for early surgery or catheter intervention.
- Understanding of cardiovascular physiology and postnatal adaptation is essential.

Examples of high-risk lesions requiring delivery at a high-level neonatal unit or cardiac centre are shown in Table 9.3.

- For many cardiac lesions, delivery can be safely planned locally, including VSDs and AVSDs, as the infant is likely to be asymptomatic in the early neonatal period.
- In this group, spontaneous onset of labour, local delivery, and postnatal cardiac review is preferred.
- There are a number of lesions where the management depends on individual features (e.g. coarctation of the aorta and tetralogy of Fallot).
- In some of these cases with 'favourable' anatomy, delivery may be planned locally but in others, cardiac support/intervention may be likely early in the neonatal period and delivery planned at a high-level centre.

Table 9.3 Factors affecting site of delivery in high-risk CHD lesions

Lesion	Concern	Risk	Delivery and management
Duct-dependent systemic blood flow, e.g. HLHS	Ductal closure Early neonatal surgery required	Cardiovascular collapse Balance of systemic and pulmonary circulation	High-level neonatal unit/cardiac centre PGE infusion
Duct-dependent pulmonary blood flow, e.g. pulmonary atresia	Ductal closure Early neonatal surgery required	Severe hypoxia	High-level neonatal intensive care unit/cardiac centre PGE infusion
Impaired mixing, e.g. TGA	Severe systemic hypoxia	Hypoxia, acidosis, death	High-level neonatal intensive care unit/cardiac centre, PGE infusion, septostomy

Table 9.4 CHD lesions that may require a planned Caesarean delivery at a cardiac centre

Lesion	Rationale
HLHS with near-intact atrial septum	Early septostomy/surgery
Severe Ebstein's anomaly	Intubation/ventilation/inhaled nitric oxide/drainage of effusions
TGA with restrictive septum	Urgent septostomy
Hydropic fetus with CHD/arrhythmia	Drainage of effusions/cardioversion

In a minority of cardiac lesions, the newborn infant may be anticipated to be critically unwell immediately after birth. These cases typically require a planned Caesarean delivery at a cardiac centre with a team immediately available. See Table 9.4.

Mode of delivery
- The diagnosis of CHD does not impact the planned mode of delivery in the vast majority of cases.
- Exceptions include the critical groups outlined above and uncontrolled arrhythmias (e.g. tachycardia/heart block) where it may be impossible to monitor fetal well-being during labour.
- The final decision is made by obstetricians taking account of all factors.

Timing of delivery
- Delivery of the fetus with CHD is generally planned at term.
- Recent guidelines caution against delivery before 39 weeks solely for cardiac reasons.
- For infants local to the cardiac centre, spontaneous onset of labour may be preferred.
- There are few indications for preterm delivery but occasionally fetuses with Ebstein's anomaly may be delivered preterm to cause a fall in PVR, or refractory arrhythmias (e.g. atrial flutter), where delivery can facilitate direct current (DC) cardioversion.

Other considerations
- It is important to consider the individual circumstance of each family, parental wishes, and wider obstetric management as well as the nature of the CHD in formulating a delivery plan.
- This will involve ongoing discussions with parents, obstetricians, fetal medicine specialists, and nurse specialists to optimize care.

Paediatric arrhythmia

Sinus tachycardia

Sinus tachycardia is common in childhood and may be misdiagnosed as a true tachyarrhythmia – or a tachyarrhythmia may be mistaken for sinus tachycardia.

Look for aetiology:
- Pain, infection, fever, dehydration, thyrotoxicosis, anaemia, heart failure, etc. should be excluded or treated.
- Monitor response to treatment.

If persistent and unexplained 'sinus' tachycardia:
- Careful review of P-wave morphology, axis, and heart rate variability is needed with a high index of suspicion in order not to miss atrial ectopic tachycardias or permanent junctional reciprocating tachycardia (PJRT) (see p. 205).
- Special caution if the history or examination is consistent with an incipient onset of heart failure, which can be secondary to tachycardia-induced cardiomyopathy.
- Rarely adenosine may be needed to distinguish between sinus and pathological tachycardias.

Supraventricular tachycardia

Supraventricular tachycardia

The term supraventricular tachycardia (SVT) covers a variety of tachycardias which originate entirely in the atrium (atrial tachycardias) or involve both atrial tissue and the AVN tissue as a critical part of a re-entry circuit (re-entry tachycardias). The majority will present as a narrow complex tachycardia (but can be broad in some circumstances).

Re-entry tachycardias

- Due to a re-entry circuit involving both the atrium and the AVN.
- There are several types of re-entry tachycardia:

Atrioventricular nodal re-entry tachycardia (AVNRT)

- Dependent on *dual AVN physiology*, in which the conduction through the AVN shows two distinct pathways with different conduction properties, typically with a *slow* and *fast* pathway.
- These provide a substrate for a re-entry tachycardia which typically passes antegrade down the slow pathway and retrograde (back to depolarize atrial tissue) via a fast pathway (Fig. 10.1).
- Therefore, in typical AVNRT there is a very short interval from the QRS to the next P wave (short RP interval).
- ECG showing pseudo-r' pattern in V1 (short RP tachycardia) (Fig. 10.2).

AVNRT:

Typical (slow–fast)

Atypical (fast–slow)

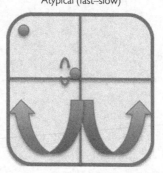

Fig. 10.1 AVNRT anatomy.

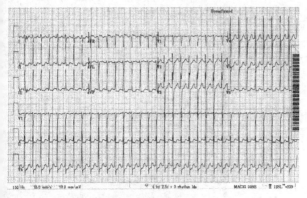

Fig. 10.2 Short RP tachycardia ECG.

Atrioventricular re-entry tachycardia (AVRT)

- Dependent on an accessory pathway providing an electrical (myocardial) bridge between the atrium and the ventricle. The AVN is a critical part of the circuit. See Fig. 10.3.
- *Typical (orthodromic) AVRT* presents as a regular, narrow complex tachycardia with short RP interval. It uses the accessory pathway as the retrograde limb of the circuit (atrium, AVN, His–Purkinje, ventricle, accessory pathway, and return to atrium).
- *Atypical (antidromic) AVRT* uses the accessory pathway as the antegrade limb, therefore depolarizing the ventricle from an ectopic focus resulting in a broad complex tachycardia, and the AVN as the retrograde pathway.

AVRT (including WPW):

Orthodromic (usual)   Antidromic (rare)

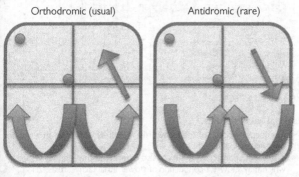

Fig. 10.3 AVRT anatomy.

Permanent junctional reciprocating tachycardia (PJRT)

- An uncommon form of AVRT with an atypical accessory pathway which conducts slowly, presenting with a typical ECG appearance of a long RP tachycardia with deeply negative P waves in the inferior leads, which can be mistaken for T-wave inversion (Fig. 10.4).
- Can be incessant and difficult to treat.
- ECG showing long RP tachycardia with deep, negative P waves in inferior leads (Fig. 10.5).

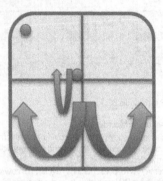

Fig. 10.4 PJRT anatomy.

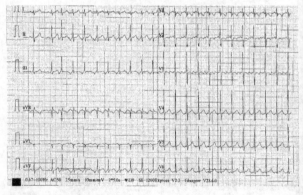

Fig. 10.5 PJRT ECG.

Atrial tachycardias

- The focus or circuit of the tachycardia is entirely within the atria and not dependent on the AVN.
- The conduction across the AVN also determines the ventricular rate, which may show 1:1 conduction of slower atrial tachycardias, 2:1 conduction, or variable conduction with irregular RR intervals.

- Adenosine may be helpful in diagnosis, by revealing the underlying atrial rhythm during the transient block of the AVN (but can also terminate the tachycardia).

There are several types of atrial tachycardia:

Atrial ectopic tachycardia

- A focal tachycardia, originating from an ectopic atrial pacemaker with automatic properties. See Fig. 10.6.
- More common in neonates.
- ECG in tachycardia would typically show a narrow complex, long RP tachycardia.
- An ECG following adenosine is shown in Fig. 10.7.
- If unrecognised and incessant can lead to a tachycardiomyopathy.

Atrial ectopic tachycardia

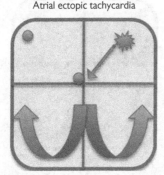

Fig. 10.6 Atrial ectopic tachycardia anatomy.

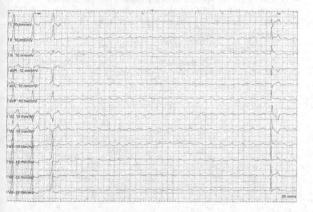

Fig. 10.7 ECG of atrial ectopic tachycardia following adenosine.

Multi-focal atrial ectopic tachycardia

Less common and presents with irregular, even chaotic atrial rhythms with multiple P-wave morphologies indicating different atrial foci.

Atrial flutter

- A macro-re-entry tachycardia within the atrium (Fig. 10.8).
- Classically presents in the antenatal period or in newborns with structurally normal hearts.
- Atypical or more complex forms of macro-re-entry atrial tachycardias are more common in older children and structural heart disease, with postoperative scar tissue often forming the substrate for an isthmus of slow conduction.

Atrial flutter

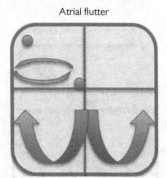

Fig. 10.8 Atrial flutter anatomy.

- 12-lead ECG in atrial flutter typically shows a narrow complex tachycardia with 2:1 AV conduction, resulting in ventricular rate of around 150 bpm. ECG following adenosine reveals typical 'sawtooth' flutter waves (Fig. 10.9).

Atrial fibrillation (AF)

Rare in children. Can be associated with CHD, inherited channelopathies, or Wolff–Parkinson–White (WPW) syndrome.

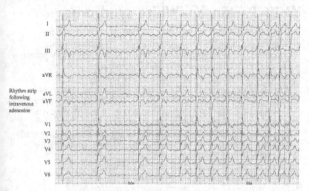

Fig. 10.9 Atrial flutter ECG.

Presentation of tachycardia

Children will present in different ways, dependent on age and underlying mechanism of arrhythmia. Older children with re-entry tachycardias typically complain of sudden-onset palpitations, which precede associated symptoms such as presyncope and chest discomfort. Neonates and pre-verbal children may present with sudden collapse, or more incipient symptoms secondary to tachycardia-induced cardiomyopathy (particularly in incessant tachycardias such as PJRT or AET).

Diagnostic clues in narrow complex tachycardias

- 12-lead ECGs in SVT should be carefully analysed:
  1. *Ventricular rate*: in re-entry tachycardias, AVRT typically presents with higher rates than AVNRT.
  2. *Regular or irregular RR intervals*: re-entry tachycardias are usually regular. Atrial tachycardias often have irregular RR intervals.
  3. *RP interval*: this describes the time interval between the QRS complex and the subsequent P wave in tachycardia. Narrow complex tachycardias can then be split into short or long RP tachycardias, describing a P seen in the first or second half of the RR interval respectively:
     a. Short RP: AVRT, typical AVNRT.
     b. Long RP: atrial tachycardia, PJRT, or rarely atypical AVNRT.
  4. *Response to adenosine*: re-entry tachycardias using the AVN as a critical part of the circuit should be terminated (at least temporarily) by adenosine. PJRT will usually be terminated, but restart. Atrial tachycardias will typically be revealed when the AVN is blocked and tachycardia continues; however, AET may also be sensitive to adenosine, with some terminating and others transiently slowed before then gradually increasing in rate back into tachycardia.
  5. *Comparison with ECG in sinus rhythm*: review for evidence of delta wave (suggesting AVRT in WPW syndrome) and pay attention to V1 in AVNRT, which may show pseudo-r′ pattern in tachycardia, but not in sinus.

Wolff–Parkinson–White syndrome

- The term Wolff–Parkinson–White (WPW) *syndrome* should be reserved for those children with ventricular pre-excitation *and* symptoms (namely palpitations and syncope), whereas WPW *pattern* can used to describe those who are asymptomatic.
- WPW syndrome is found in around 1–3 in 1000 in the general population (first-degree relatives have a slightly higher incidence).
- Ventricular pre-excitation is caused by an 'accessory pathway' providing a myocardial bridge (crossing the fibrous rings of the AV valves) which allows conduction between the atrium and ventricle.
- Ventricular pre-excitation is manifested by a short PR interval, slurred upstroke or downstroke to QRS (the 'delta wave'), with widening of the QRS complex.

WPW predisposes to several arrhythmias:
- *Orthodromic AVRT*: should be managed as any other AVRT.
- *Antidromic AVRT*: presents as a broad complex tachycardia.
- *Pre-excited AF*: if the accessory pathway is able to conduct rapidly in the antegrade direction, pre-excited AF (an irregular broad complex tachycardia) may lead to a rapid ventricular rate and even *ventricular fibrillation* (the presumed mechanism for a higher incidence of sudden cardiac death (SCD) seen in patients with WPW). Malignant arrhythmias can be the sentinel symptom in WPW.
- The accessory pathway is also able to act as a *bystander* in other arrhythmias (such as AVNRT) and not participate in the tachycardia.

Treatment and risk stratification

- *WPW syndrome*: symptoms (typically due to orthodromic AVRT) can be managed medically in younger children. Beta-blockers are commonly used and appear safe in orthodromic AVRT, where as flecainide would be preferred in antidromic AVRT to better target AP conduction. Drugs that primarily slow AV node conduction (adenosine, beta-blockers, verapamil and digoxin) should be avoided in pre-excited AF (due to the risk of slowing AVN conduction and promoting rapid conduction via the accessory pathway). Children 4–5 years of age or older (>15–20 kg) may be referred for consideration of catheter ablation.
- *WPW pattern*: no antiarrhythmic medication required. Can still be considered for invasive EP study (usually above 5 years), outlining the balance of the procedural risk versus the albeit low, lifetime risk of malignant arrhythmias.

Management of supraventricular tachycardia

Acute treatment

- Acute management of SVT should be based on national paediatric resuscitation guidelines.
- Initial systematic assessment of the child determines whether they are *haemodynamically compromised*, requiring support from anaesthetic or ICU colleagues to stabilize and then deliver prompt synchronised DC cardioversion to restore sinus rhythm.
- Most children tolerate surprisingly long periods in SVT and a calm, systematic approach to diagnosis and management should be taken:
  - *Vagal manoeuvres* followed, if needed, by adenosine administration should be undertaken with a rhythm strip running (at least three and up to 12 leads if possible).
  - *Adenosine* administration is generally safe in children; however, it should always be performed with suitable resuscitation equipment available as on rare occasions it can accelerate a tachycardia. Caution should be taken in children with known severe asthma or sinus node dysfunction and it is contraindicated in pre-excited AF.
  - *Amiodarone* may be required in refractory SVT, but should be used cautiously and after expert advice.

Long-term management of paroxysmal SVT

Paroxysmal SVT in older children with normal heart structure and function is generally a benign arrhythmia. Treatment strategies should therefore be primarily dictated by the frequency and severity of the child's symptoms. Treatment options fall broadly into the following:

- *Conservative treatment*: outside of neonatal period, in paroxysmal SVT without collapse, a strategy of no treatment and continued monitoring for burden of symptoms is reasonable.
- *Regular antiarrhythmic medication*: daily medication can reduce burden of symptoms. For neonatal SVT, it is reasonable to treat with medications until 6–12 months of age, before stopping after the child has outgrown the medication dose.
- *EP study and ablation*: definitive treatment option increasingly favoured in children for recurrent SVT, usually above the age of 4–5 years, or 15 kg (see p. 167).

Antiarrhythmic medication options (see pharmacology section)

- Beta-blockers remain the first-line treatment for a majority of SVT. Propranolol often used in neonatal period with conversion to longer-acting agent in infancy and older (atenolol or bisoprolol).
- Flecainide is commonly relied on as a second-line agent, almost always in combination with AVN-slowing agent such as a beta-blocker. It is helpful in a variety of SVT, slowing accessory pathway conduction in AVRT and reducing ectopy in automatic tachycardias (such as atrial ectopic tachycardia). It should be used with caution in children with structural heart disease.

Ventricular tachycardia

VT is relatively rare in children, with an incidence of around 1 in 100,000 patient years. Causes include CHD, myocarditis, inherited arrhythmias (such as LQTS and CPVT), cardiomyopathies (such as HCM and ARVC), and ischaemic cardiomyopathy. Compared to adults, 'idiopathic' and usually benign VT makes up a far larger proportion of VT cases.

> Neither the rate nor clinical presentation are enough to distinguish between SVT and VT. How unwell the child is depends on both the rate of the tachycardia and its duration.

Diagnosis

A structured approach should be taken to analyse ECGs of children presenting in stable broad complex tachycardias as over half may represent SVT with rate-related or pre-existing bundle branch block. *Features suggesting VT* (rather than SVT) include the following:

- *VA dissociation*: with more QRS complexes than P waves is diagnostic.
- *Capture or fusion beats*: representing sinus node 'capture' of ventricle via normal antegrade conduction down the His–Purkinje system.
- *Concordance in precordial leads*: all leads V1–6 showing either predominantly positive or negative QRS complexes (whereas more typical RBBB or LBBB more common in SVT with aberrancy).
- *QRS width*: very broad QRS complexes more likely VT; adult data suggests >140 msec in RBBB and >160 msec in LBBB.
- *QRS axis*: paediatric data showing left, superior axis deviation more commonly associated with VT (commonly fascicular VT).
- *Use of adenosine*: in a stable child presenting in a *regular* broad complex tachycardia, adenosine should be used to help distinguish SVT from VT and may give diagnostic information (e.g. reveal temporary VA dissociation in VT with 1:1 VA conduction) and can terminate a small proportion of VT.

Management

Similar to SVT, the initial management of VT should be based on national Advanced Paediatric Life Support algorithms for broad complex tachycardia with assessment of haemodynamic status and prompt synchronised DC cardioversion in collapsed patients. Specific examples with management strategies are discussed below.

Fascicular ventricular tachycardia

- Also known as 'verapamil-sensitive VT'.
- A re-entry tachycardia around the Purkinje fibres of the fascicles.
- 90% arise from the left posterior fascicle, presenting with a RBBB pattern with left/superior axis (± other features of VT, such as VA dissociation or capture beats).
- Uniquely sensitive to calcium channel blockers with >90% cardioversion rates with verapamil.

- Verapamil should be used only with extreme caution in children <1 year of age due to concerns of irreversible haemodynamic collapse.
- Typically presents as a refractory "SVT" (apparently not responsive to adenosine, nor initial treatment with amiodarone).
- Radiofrequency ablation has good success rates.

RVOT ventricular tachycardia

- The RVOT is one of the most common origins of monomorphic premature ventricular complexes and sustained VT in children with structurally normal hearts.
- Monomorphic premature ventricular complexes from RVOT in children are common and usually benign; however, paediatric data suggest that >30% burden of premature ventricular complexes can be associated with LV dysfunction and sustained VT.
- RVOT VT is often induced with exercise or adrenergic drive.
- Characterized by LBBB pattern and inferior axis.
- May terminate with adenosine.
- Acute treatment includes DC cardioversion, esmolol, and lidocaine.
- Long-term treatment includes beta-blockers and catheter ablation.

Bradycardias

Bradycardias are defined as heart rates below the normal limits for age (see p. 321). As an incidental finding in otherwise well children, they are a surprisingly common cause for referral and are usually benign. They should prompt review and documentation of heart rhythm on a 12-lead ECG. History should focus on cardiac symptoms (e.g. syncope and exercise intolerance) and systemic symptoms, such as lethargy or a prodrome suggestive of infection. Past medical history of CHD, metabolic and endocrine disorders, as well as eating disorders in older children are relevant.

Sinus bradycardia

- If persistent and pronounced should prompt further investigations for underlying causes, including hypothyroidism, drugs (e.g. beta-blockers, opioids), hypothermia, electrolyte abnormalities, and raised intracranial pressure.
- *Sinus node dysfunction* is rare in children, in the absence of CHD or inherited arrhythmias (e.g. LQTS, or Brugada syndrome). It is more commonly seen in older children, or young adults, following surgery for CHD (e.g. Fontan or atrial switch procedures).

Junctional bradycardia

Can be observed in otherwise healthy children at rest, or at night, is usually transient, and will be suppressed by increasing sinus rates with activity.

Atrioventricular block

First-degree AV block

- PR interval ≥ upper limits for age.
- Can be normal variant, but positive history (e.g. cardiac syncope) or family history should prompt further investigations or period of monitoring.

Second-degree AV block

- Mobitz I pattern (AV Wenckebach):
  - Progressive PR prolongation, followed by non-conducted P wave.
  - Usually a benign finding.
- Mobitz II pattern:
  - Intermittent non-conducted P-waves, without PR prolongation, fixed ratio (2:1, 3:1).
  - Abnormal, can progress to complete heart block.

Third-degree (complete) heart block

- Abnormal, requires review by a paediatric cardiologist.
- Although congenital AV block is the most common form of complete heart block, a first presentation particularly in older children should consider other causes, such as CHD (e.g. ccTGA), infectious triggers (e.g. myocarditis, Lyme disease, rheumatic fever), and others (autoimmune, metabolic, and neuromuscular diseases and channelopathies associated with conduction disease).

Bradycardias in special circumstances

- *Newborns*: initial assessment of neonatal bradycardia (≤90 bpm), a common clinical scenario, should focus on:
  - Premature atrial ectopic beats with compensatory sinus pauses
  - Congenital AV block
  - QT interval (LQTS can present with fetal and neonatal sinus bradycardia, as well as functional 2:1 block in neonates with significantly prolonged QT interval).
- *Postoperative*: both sinus node and AVN dysfunction can occur following surgery for CHD. Epicardial pacing wires are used in anticipation of postoperative rhythm disturbances, which are often transient.

Pacing and pacemakers in children

Permanent cardiac pacing in children is challenging due to patient size, an anticipated lifetime requirement for pacing, and, in the context of CHB, anatomical considerations requiring individualized lead placements. The indications for permanent pacing in children should be balanced, taking into account not only the acute procedural risks (i.e. pneumothorax or lead displacement), but the ongoing risks of infection, lead malfunction, venous obstruction, and the need for lead extraction.

Indications

The most common indications for pacemaker implantation in children are:

Congenital complete heart block (CCHB)

- CCHB in newborn or infant with symptomatic bradycardia, or asymptomatic with ventricular rate <50bpm (or <60-70bpm with associated CHD).
- CCHB with wide complex escape rhythm, complex ventricular ectopy, or ventricular dysfunction.
- CCHB beyond first year of life with average ventricular rate <50 bpm, abrupt pauses, or symptoms of chronotropic incompetence.

Other childhood-onset heart block

- Advanced second- or third-degree AV block with symptoms of chronotropic incompetence, ventricular dysfunction, or low cardiac output.

Postoperative heart block

- Advanced second- or third-degree AV block not expected to resolve or persisting at least 7 days after cardiac surgery.

Other indications

- Sinus node dysfunction (bradycardia <40bpm or pauses >3 seconds) and correlating with symptoms).
- Combination of tachyarrhythmias requiring antiarrhythmic medication and sinus node dysfunction.
- Neuromuscular diseases associated with conduction disease.
- Neurocardiogenic syncope (rarely indicated, and only when severe symptoms correlated with cardioinhibitory response on ambulatory ECG or tilt test).

System choice

- In smaller children, there is little advantage in AV-synchronous pacing, therefore commonly a single-chamber (VVI) device is selected until the child is older (>20 kg), when generator changes can be combined with addition of atrial lead for dual-chamber pacing.
- Epicardial leads are generally favoured in small children (<10 kg particularly), where endocardial access is limited (i.e. Fontan circulation), or for postoperative complete heart block (depending on patient factors).

Pacing modes

Standardized codes used with four positions, listed in order of:
1. Chamber paced (A = atrium, V = ventricle, D = dual)
2. Chamber sensed (A = atrium, V = ventricle, D = dual)
3. Response to sensing (T = triggered, I = inhibited, D = dual)
4. Rate modulation (R = rate responsive).

Common examples and indications are listed below:

VVI/VVIR
- Single-chamber pacing.
- Paces and senses ventricle only and inhibits pacing if intrinsic QRS sensed above base rate (therefore allowing intrinsic rhythm where appropriate).
- Rate response programmed to increase base rate when activity sensed.
- Example of use: small children with CCHB.

AAI/AAIR
- Single-chamber pacing.
- Paces and senses atria only, inhibits if intrinsic P wave sensed.
- Can have rate response programmed to increase base rate when activity sensed.
- Used for sinus node dysfunction, but preserved AV conduction (e.g. post-Fontan or atrial switch operation).

DDD
- Dual-chamber pacing.
- Paces and senses both atria and ventricles.
- Response to sensing is 'dual', meaning it inhibits in either chamber if intrinsic P wave or QRS complex is detected, but also allows AV synchrony by tracking intrinsic P waves and pacing ventricle after defined AV delay.
- Rate response (DDDR) only indicated with additional sinus node dysfunction.
- Commonly used in older children with congenital or acquired AV block.

Channelopathies

The inherited cardiac ion 'channelopathies' represent an important cause of SCD in children and young adults, also referred to as 'sudden arrhythmogenic death syndrome'.

Long QT syndrome

- The LQTS has an prevalence of 1:2000, and predisposes individuals to a risk of malignant ventricular arrhythmias (torsade des pointes) and sudden death.
- It must be considered after exclusion of reversible causes of QT prolongation which lead to *acquired* long QT interval.
- Presentations typically include syncope, or aborted SCD, after family screening or as an incidental finding.

Genetic basis

- As research into the genetic basis of LQTS continues to evolve, there are now 16 subtypes described; however, ~20% of cases remain genetically elusive.
- Of genotype-positive patients, a majority (90%) are caused by mutations in three genes, causing three distinct subtypes of LQTS: *KCNQ1* (causing LQT1), *KCNH2* (causing LQT2) or *SCN5A* (causing LQT3). The remaining 10% are caused by the 'minor' LQTS genes.
- A majority are inherited in an autosomal dominant pattern (so-called Romano–Ward syndrome) with no extracardiac features.
- Rare subtypes are important to recognize with a high burden of arrhythmias:
  - A severe autosomal recessive form of LQTS (Jervell and Lange-Nielson syndrome) is associated with congenital deafness.
  - Two rare forms of LQTS exist with multisystem involvement and typical constellation of extracardiac features (Andersen–Tawil syndrome and Timothy syndrome).
  - More recently three subtypes of LQTS have been described with affected genes encoding calmodulin protein (CALM1–3), with sporadic inheritance pattern and a severe clinical course.

Calculating the corrected QT interval

The Bazett formula (QT/square root of preceding RR interval in lead II or V5) using the tangent method is recommended (Fig. 10.10).

Once the QTc is carefully calculated (ideally averaged across three consecutive beats in leads II or V5), the data can be inputted into the website www.QTcalculator.org, which provides the probability of LQTS in the patient (suggesting a conservative cut-off of the 99th centile in the control population).

Diagnosis

In all cases, reversible causes of QT prolongation should be excluded (consider electrolyte disturbances, QT-prolonging drugs, and hypothermia).

LQTS can be diagnosed when:

- QTc >480 ms in repeated ECGs in asymptomatic individual, *or*
- QTc of >460 ms in a patient with arrhythmic syncope, *or*
- There is a pathogenic mutation in long QT gene, *or*
- A long QT diagnostic score >3 (Table 10.1).

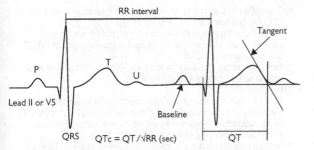

Fig. 10.10 Tangent method measuring QTc.

Reprinted from Postema, P.G., et al (2008) Accurate electrocardiographic assessment of the QT interval: teach the tangent. Heart Rhythm 5(7):1015–18.

Table 10.1 Modified long QT syndrome diagnostic score

Features	Points
Electrocardiographic findings	
– A QTc interval (using Bazett formula):	
≥480 ms	3.5
460–479 ms	2
450–459 ms (in males)	1
– QTc >480 ms during 4th minute of recovery from exercise stress test	1
– Documented torsades de pointes	2
– T wave alternans	1
– Notched T wave in three leads	1
– Low heart rate for age	0.5
Clinical history	
– Syncope:	
With stress	2
Without stress	1
Family history	
– Relatives with clinically definitive LQTS	1
– Unexplained SCD in immediate relative <30 years	0.5
Genetic testing	
– Pathogenic mutation	3.5

Management

The diagnosis and management of children with LQTS should be led by experienced clinicians. Management strategies include the following:
- *Lifestyle advice:*
  - Avoid medicines known to prolong QT interval, which can be found at www.crediblemeds.org.

* Correction of electrolyte disturbances that may occur during periods of illness (such as diarrhoea and vomiting).
* Avoid triggers for arrhythmias, specific to genotype, such as (unsupervised) swimming and high-level competitive sports in LQT1 and loud alarms in LQT2.
* Family members of children and adults with inherited arrhythmias should be trained in basic life support.

* *Medication:*
  * Beta-blockers are recommended in anyone with symptoms, and those meeting unequivocal diagnostic criteria of LQTS, and should be considered in asymptomatic individuals with pathogenic gene mutations, even in the presence of a normal QTc.
  * Sodium channel blockers (such as mexiletine or flecainide) should be considered to reduce QT interval in children with LQT3 and QTc >500 ms.

* *Implantable cardioverter defibrillators* (ICDs):
  * Recommended in patients with LQTS and previous cardiac arrest.
  * Considered in patients with LQTS with syncope and/or VT despite adequate treatment with beta-blockers.
  * Should be considered in asymptomatic patients felt to be at particularly high risk.

* *Left cardiac sympathetic denervation* may be considered in high-risk patients, or those with recurrent arrhythmias despite optimal medical management.

Brugada syndrome

Brugada syndrome is a cause of SCD in the young. It is uncommon, with a prevalence of around 1-2 per 10,000 in Europe, but higher in Asian countries. It is more common in males.

Presentation

The first presentation may be SCD or aborted SCD, commonly during sleep or at rest. It usually presents in the third decade of life but is also seen in children. Many patients are asymptomatic, and more children and adults are now diagnosed due to family screening.

Investigation and diagnostic criteria

There is no gold standard investigation for diagnosis and family screening in asymptomatic individuals can be challenging. It is commonly diagnosed by:

* ST-segment elevation with type 1 morphology (see example in Fig. 10.11) with ≥2 mm in one or more leads among the right precordial leads V1, V2, positioned in the second, third, or fourth intercostal space occurring either spontaneously or after provocative drug test with IV administration of class I antiarrhythmic drugs.

* Performing a 15-lead (or 'high-lead') ECG can unmask spontaneous type 1 pattern in children with Brugada syndrome. This is achieved by moving V1, V2, and V3 electrodes above their standard positions (or adding additional electrodes) to the third (or second) intercostal space.

* IV ajmaline (a sodium channel blocker) can also be used to unmask a type 1 Brugada pattern. This should only be performed in an experienced centre following adequate counselling of the child and

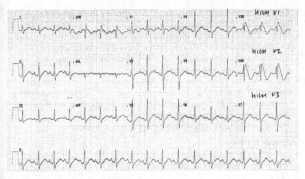

Fig. 10.11 ECG of type 1 Brugada.

family of its risks (provoking ventricular arrhythmias) and prognostic use. It is a useful, but imperfect test which is routinely left until the teenage years because after puberty it may become positive in up to 23% when previously negative earlier in childhood.

- Genetics may be helpful in some cases but are probabilistic only and challenging to interpret. The most common genetic variant seen involves the sodium channel gene *SCN5A*. However, *SCN5A* has common variants in the general population and in some families the phenotype does not segregate with the genotype.

Management

- Avoid drugs listed on www.brugadadrugs.org.
- Manage febrile illnesses with antipyretics and avoid dehydration.
- Fevers not responding to simple measures should prompt review in hospital for diagnostic ECG performed *during* fever (as febrile illness may unmask Brugada pattern) and to monitor for arrhythmias, particularly in smaller children with confirmed diagnosis.
- Older children and young adults should be advised to avoid alcohol excess or large meals prior to sleeping (related to vagal tone).
- ICD implantation remains the only method of preventing SCD in children with Brugada syndrome but is not without complications in children.
- Quinidine may be useful for recurrent arrhythmias to prevent ICD discharges or where an ICD is not used.
- Isoprenaline can be helpful in acute treatment of arrhythmia storms in Brugada syndrome.

Catecholaminergic polymorphic ventricular tachycardia (CPVT)

- Rare inherited cardiac channelopathy with a prevalence estimated at around 1 in 10,000.
- Although uncommon, it represents an important cause of SCD in the young.

- Typically present with symptoms of syncope or cardiac arrest on exercise or with emotional stress.
- A high index of suspicion therefore required for symptoms on exercise or stress in presence of *normal* resting ECG and echocardiogram.
- Exercise stress test-induced (see p. 101) ventricular arrhythmias is diagnostic in the otherwise normal heart.
- Genetic mutations found in up to 70% of patients, most affecting three genes: *RYR2* (majority of mutations), *CASQ2*, and *TRDN*, which together encode proteins of the ryanodine channel complex, involved in calcium release from sarcoplasmic reticulum.
- Probands may have higher incidence of lethal arrhythmias.

Diagnostic criteria

- Exercise or emotion-induced bidirectional (Fig. 10.12) or polymorphic VT (in the presence of a structurally normal heart with normal resting ECG).
- Presence of pathogenic genetic mutation(s) in the *RYR2* or *CASQ2* genes.

Management

- High-dose beta-blockers remain the first-line treatment.
- Flecainide has been shown to be a particularly effective second-line medical treatment.
- Strict compliance is essential, use ECG and exercise ECG to monitor response.
- Avoid triggers (both emotional and exercise).
- ICD indicated in the setting of recurrent syncope, aborted SCD or bidirectional/polymorphic VT despite adequate treatment.
- Left cardiac sympathetic denervation can be considered in patients with recurrent symptoms or appropriate ICD shocks, despite optimal medical therapy.

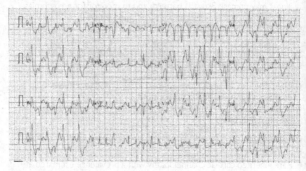

Fig. 10.12 ECG of bidirectional VT in CPVT.

Heart muscle disease and cardiac transplantation

Cardiomyopathies

Cardiomyopathies are myocardial disorders in which the heart muscle is structurally and functionally abnormal (in the absence of a factor sufficiently severe to cause the observed myocardial abnormality, such as coronary artery disease, hypertension, valvular disease, or CHD).

Dilated cardiomyopathy (DCM)

DCM is the common end point of a wide range of heterogeneous conditions, rather than a single disease. A detailed family history should be taken to help identify a genetic cause (history of SCD, pacemaker insertion, strokes at a young age, muscular weakness, and autoimmune disease).

Causes

A specific cause is identified in only 30–40% of cases (Table 11.1), the rest are classified as idiopathic.

Table 11.1 Causes of DCM in children

Genetic—autosomal dominant	Dystrophinopathies, e.g. Duchenne/Becker muscular dystrophy
	Nuclear membrane, e.g. lamin A/C mutation, Emery Dreifuss muscular dystrophy
	Sarcomeric protein, e.g. MYH7, TTN, TNNT2, TPM1, troponin I/C, MYL2
	Cytoskeletal protein, e.g. desmin
	Ion channel protein genes or Ca^{2+} regulation, e.g. SCN5A
	Other, e.g. BAG3, RBM20, filamin C (FLNC)
Genetic—X-linked	Dystrophinopathies, e.g. Duchenne/Becker muscular dystrophy
	Glycogen storage diseases, e.g. Danon (LAMP2 mutations)
	Barth syndrome (TAZ mutations)
Genetic—mitochondrial	Mitochondrial cytopathy (mitochondrial inheritance), e.g. Kearns–Sayre, MELAS, MERRF
Infectious	Viral, bacterial, fungal, protozoal (Chagas, toxoplasmosis), rickettsia (Rocky Mountain spotted fever), spirochaetal (Lyme disease)
Toxins	Anthracyclines, radiation, other chemotherapeutic agents, sulphonamide sensitivity, penicillin sensitivity, iron (haemochromatosis), copper (Wilson's disease)
Nutritional	Protein (kwashiorkor), thiamine (beriberi), vitamin E, vitamin D, selenium, carnitine (deficiency or transporter defects), phosphate

Table 11.1 (Contd.)

Systemic	Systemic lupus erythematosus, juvenile idiopathic arthritis, polyarteritis nodosa, osteogenesis imperfecta, Noonan syndrome, peripartum cardiomyopathy, haemolytic uraemic syndrome, leukaemia, amyloidosis, sarcoidosis, Reye syndrome
Arrhythmia	Tachycardiomyopathy
Endocrine	Thyroid disorders, catecholamine excess (phaeochromocytoma or neuroblastoma), congenital adrenal hyperplasia
Ischaemia	Hypoxia, birth asphyxia, drowning, KD, coronary artery malformation (ALCAPA), premature coronary artery disease

Prevalence

Most common form of heart muscle disease in children, although still rare: 0.6–0.8/100,000 children. May occur at any age.

Clinical features

- Severity varies, from mild and slowly progressing disease to fulminant heart failure.
- Onset usually gradual, with vague long-standing symptoms.
- Clinical signs are those of 'pump failure' (see p. 15).
- Causes listed in Table 11.1 may have specific symptoms and signs in addition to those of heart failure.

Investigation

At first presentation a wide-ranging panel of investigations should be undertaken, aiming to identify potentially reversible causes (Table 11.2).

CXR

- Cardiomegaly, possibly with signs of pulmonary oedema.

ECG

- Sinus tachycardia.
- Non-specific ST and T-wave changes.
- Atrial enlargement.
- Ventricular hypertrophy.

TTE

- It is important to demonstrate that the heart is structurally normal, including coronary anatomy.
- Dilated LV, with biventricular or atrial enlargement in some advanced cases.
- May be RV involvement and/or diastolic dysfunction.
- Complications of DCM such as intracardiac thrombus may be seen.

Table 11.2 Example first-line investigation screening panel for DCM

Echocardiogram	Bloods
ECG, including 24-hour tape	FBC
CXR	Erythrocyte sedimentation rate
Urine	Vacuolated lymphocytes
Organic acids	U&E
Glycosaminoglycans	LFTs
	C-reactive protein
	Brain natriuretic peptide
	Blood group and save
	Lactate
	Ammonia
	Cholesterol and triglycerides
	Thyroid function tests
	Thiamine
	Selenium
	Red blood cell transketolase
	Carnitine
	Acyl carnitine profile
	Red cell folate
	Transferrin
	Mitochondrial DNA
	Plasma amino acids
	Antinuclear and anti-DNA antibodies
	Viral PCR, immunoglobulin (Ig)-M and IgG for enterovirus, Epstein–Barr virus, adenovirus, cytomegalovirus, parvovirus, coxsackievirus, echovirus
	Ionized calcium
	Parathyroid hormone
	Vitamin D

Additional tests may be required depending on the nature of the initial presentation

Ambulatory ECG
- May identify arrhythmias as a primary cause (or poorly tolerated complication) of DCM.
- The presence of malignant arrhythmias may indicate the need for specific treatment.

Cardiac MRI
- May further characterize myocardial abnormalities.

Endomyocardial biopsy
- Not usually performed in the UK for diagnostic purposes in the setting of DCM/myocarditis, as it is felt the risks do not outweigh the benefits.
- In addition, myocarditis has been shown to attack the myocardium in a patchy fashion, increasing the chance of a false negative if healthy myocardium is sampled.

Management
Directed at addressing both heart failure and the underlying cause (see p. 224).

Outcome
The 5-year freedom from death or transplantation is 54–63%. The main predictor is degree of LV dysfunction at presentation.

Myocarditis

Although usually considered a separate disease entity to DCM, infectious myocarditis is the most common cause of the DCM phenotype. The pathogenic process is not completely understood. Initial infection → inflammation and myocardial injury (cytotoxic lymphocytes attack infected cells, increasing circulating autoantibodies → dilatation of the heart, with failure of regulatory mechanisms that would normally increase force of contraction.

Causes
Most commonly viruses (enteroviruses and adenoviruses); worldwide, protozoa (in particular Chagas disease—caused by *Trypanosoma cruzi* infection) dominate.

Presentation
Enterovirus myocarditis in infants may be associated with enterovirus meningitis. In older children there may have been recent symptoms of a viral infection. These are then followed by clinical signs of 'pump failure' (see p. 15).

Prognosis
Complete resolution in up to 1/3, progression to chronic DCM in others.

Hypertrophic cardiomyopathy (HCM)

HCM is characterized by LV hypertrophy (Z score ≥2) in the absence of abnormal loading conditions (e.g. hypertension, valvular or congenital heart disease) sufficient to account for the degree of hypertrophy.

HCM is a phenotype and not a final diagnosis. The history, family, and investigations may point to a particular aetiology.

Causes
- Majority caused by sarcomeric protein gene mutations (autosomal dominant) most commonly found in *MYH7* and myosin binding protein C (*MYBPC3*) genes.
- Infants may have inborn errors of metabolism.
- Older children may have neuromuscular disease (e.g. Friedreich's ataxia).
- Genotype–phenotype correlations have been reported but genetic testing does not currently affect management. Its main role is to allow for cascade family screening.

Prevalence
- Rare in children, 0.24–0.47 per 100,000.

Clinical features
- *Infants*: more likely to present with symptoms of congestive cardiac failure.
- *Older children*: symptoms include those of heart failure (dyspnoea and exercise intolerance), and those of LVOTO or impaired LV diastolic function (chest pain, syncope, palpitations).

Investigations

ECG
- Abnormal in 95% and may precede development of LV hypertrophy.
- Voltage criteria for LV hypertrophy (non-specific).
- Repolarization abnormalities (e.g. inverted T waves, ST-segment abnormalities).
- Pathological Q waves.

TTE
- *Hypertrophy* (assess the extent and pattern).
- *LVOT obstruction* (maximum gradient ≥30 mmHg) is dynamic and multifactorial (basal anteroseptal hypertrophy, systolic anterior motion of mitral valve, abnormal valvar chordal attachments).
- *Diastolic function* commonly impaired.
- *Systolic function* typically 'supra-normal' (ejection fraction 60%), although in end-stage disease this falls ("burnt-out HCM").

Ambulatory ECG
- For atrial and ventricular arrhythmias, important for risk stratification of arrhythmic events.

Cardiac MRI
- LV mass, late gadolinium enhancement identifies areas of myocardial fibrosis.

Management
No medical therapy has been shown to change prognosis so treating asymptomatic obstruction is controversial. Focus is on relieving symptoms although for some inborn errors of metabolism disease specific therapy is available (e.g. enzyme replacement therapy in Pompe's disease).

Symptomatic patient with LVOTO
- Beta-blockers, disopyramide, and calcium channel blockers.
- Surgical myectomy can be used to relieve LVOT obstruction.

Symptomatic patient with no LVOTO
- Largely empirical (beta-blockers and calcium channel blockers).

Sudden cardiac death in HCM (event rate 1–2% per year)
- No medical therapy is recommended as preventative therapy.
- ICDs are used for secondary prevention following an episode of malignant arrhythmia.
- Risk factors for SCD in childhood include maximal LV wall thickness, non-sustained VT, unexplained syncope, LA diameter, and LVOT gradient.

- Validated paediatric specific risk models (e.g. HCM Risk Kids) are available to guide primary prevention ICD decision making.

Family screening
- The majority of childhood disease diagnosed through screening is diagnosed at ≤12 years of age.
- Guidelines recommend commencing screening at any age following the diagnosis of HCM in a first-degree relative.
- Clinical screening consists of history, clinical examination, ECG, and echocardiography.
- Regular clinical assessment is required throughout childhood due to variable and age-related penetrance.
- Predictive genetic testing may be possible if a disease-causing variant is identified in the family.

Outcome
Varies depending on the underlying aetiology and age of presentation. Progression to 'end-stage disease' is rare during childhood in sarcomeric disease.
- Patients with non-syndromic disease have a relatively good prognosis (5-year survival 80–85%).
- Patients with inborn errors of metabolism or malformation syndromes have a worse prognosis (1-year survival of 54% or 82%, respectively).
- Presentation in infancy is associated with a worse prognosis (1-year mortality 14%) with death most commonly secondary to heart failure. However, for those that survive to 1 year, mortality is similar to those presenting later in childhood.
- The most common cause of death, outside of infancy, is SCD.

Restrictive cardiomyopathy (RCM)

RCM is a rare form of cardiomyopathy in children. It is characterized by reduced LV compliance, resulting in diastolic dysfunction, raised LVEDP, and subsequent pulmonary hypertension. This eventually results in reduced cardiac output, and subsequent heart failure. The development of raised pulmonary pressures can be rapid or insidious, requiring early transplantation consideration. The outlook without cardiac transplantation is poor.

Cause
- Most idiopathic, although may be caused by many infiltrative and metabolic disorders. 1/3 have a clear familial pattern.

Clinical features
- Mostly relate to the resulting congestive cardiac failure.

Investigations
- CXR: may show cardiomegaly (related to atrial dilatation).
- Echocardiography: systolic function is usually normal in the initial period and diastolic function is impaired (often grossly so). Typical pattern of marked biatrial enlargement is seen (also on ECG).
- PVRi measurement in most cases is advised.

Management
No medical therapy has been shown to change prognosis. Early transplant listing is dictated by PVR.

Arrhythmogenic cardiomyopathies

Very rare in childhood but are the second commonest cause of sudden death in young adults after HCM. They include ARVC. A spectrum of clinical phenotypes exists with structural abnormalities of the myocardium (regional/global systolic dysfunction, or myocardial scar) and frequent ventricular ectopy or malignant ventricular arrhythmias.

Cause
- Familial disease with predominantly autosomal dominant inheritance.

Investigations
- ECG: repolarization abnormalities in right precordial leads, delayed depolarization, and arrhythmias.
- Echocardiography: may show RV dilatation, akinesia, or aneurysms.
- Histological (fibro-fatty replacement).

Management
- Treatment of heart failure symptoms.
- Prevention of arrhythmias with medical therapy (beta-blockers, amiodarone) and ICD implantation.
- Exercise restriction is recommended in all patients diagnosed with ARVC as exercise has been shown to cause disease progression.

Chemotherapy-induced cardiotoxicity

Cardiovascular disease is the leading contributor to morbidity and mortality in cancer survivors (eightfold higher risk of cardiovascular-related deaths when compared to healthy children).

Anthracyclines such as doxorubicin and daunorubicin are the main cardiotoxic agents. Prompt, early detection should be the primary aim as doing so allows treatment, leading to improved outcomes.

Definition

No paediatric definition, but the adult definition is a reduction in LV ejection fraction by >10% to a value of <53%. It may be *acute* (within 1 week of exposure, fully reversible with removal of the inciting agent), *early onset* (within 1 year, progressive course), or *late onset* (after >1 year, spectrum of presentation from subclinical ventricular dysfunction to overt heart failure and cardiomyopathy).

Risk factors

Higher cumulative dose of anthracycline, especially ≥300 mg/m², longer time from anthracycline treatment, concomitant radiotherapy, younger age (<4 years), trisomy 21, female sex, and genetic factors.

Echocardiography

Conventional metrics of function (ejection fraction, fractional shortening) are not sensitive in early detection of cardiotoxicity. LV strain, especially global longitudinal strain, is superior. Diastolic dysfunction precedes systolic impairment and should be evaluated. Protocols for cardiac follow-up depend on age of first treatment, concomitant radiation therapy, and cumulative dose.

Treatment

ACEi is the main class of medication used (see p. 282).

Heart failure management

Heart failure in children is a clinical syndrome resulting from ventricular dysfunction, with volume, or pressure overload, alone or in combination (see p. 12). It leads to characteristic signs and symptoms, including poor growth, feeding difficulties, respiratory distress, exercise intolerance, and fatigue, associated with circulatory, neurohormonal, and molecular abnormalities.

This section is focused on the management of heart failure secondary to heart muscle disease (for the management of heart failure secondary to congenital heart disease, see p. 13 and p. 130).

Immediate treatment focuses on resuscitation and haemodynamic stability (with ventilation and inotropes if required), followed by normalization of fluid status. When possible, patients should be transitioned to oral medications.

Diuretics

- Care must be taken to avoid over-diuresis and electrolyte imbalance (cardiac output may fall if the patient becomes fluid depleted, particularly in HCM and RCM).
- A loop diuretic is usually accompanied by spironolactone. In addition to helping normalize K$^+$ levels, it has been shown to improve survival in adults with heart failure.

Angiotensin-converting enzyme inhibitors

- Reduce SVR to improve cardiac output.
- Inhibit maladaptive compensatory mechanisms involving the renin–aldosterone–angiotensin system, slowing the rate of myocardial damage, and leading to reverse remodelling of the LV. If contraindicated, may be substituted with an angiotensin receptor blocker.
- Captopril, enalapril, and lisinopril are the most commonly used, with doses gradually titrated up, while checking for hypotension and renal impairment (both relatively rare in this group).
- Improved survival has been demonstrated in adults.

Beta-blockers

- Indicated in chronic heart failure, not in the acute phase when native sympathetic activity might still be required; accordingly, beta-blockers may need to be stopped during acute exacerbations.
- It may seem counterintuitive to slow the HR in low cardiac output, but it is felt that chronic activation of the adrenergic response leads to reduction of beta receptors and a maladaptive response, hence the beneficial effects of beta-blockade.
- Improvements in survival have been demonstrated.

Digoxin

- Positively inotropic and negatively chronotropic increases cardiac output.
- Due to potential toxicity, it must be used with caution in acutely ill children, but the reduction in HR is felt to be beneficial overall.

Anticoagulation

- Reduced systolic function and dilatation of the LV leads to additional risk of intracardiac thrombosis and subsequent stroke (usually started if fractional shortening <20%).
- Aspirin is most commonly used, though patients with existing thrombus or severely impaired function may need warfarin or unfractionated heparin.

Other treatment considerations

- Arrhythmias should be treated promptly. Resynchronization therapy with biventricular pacing may be indicated in those with significant dyssynchrony, with excellent results in some patients.
- Electrolyte imbalance should be corrected.
- Anaemia may require earlier transfusion than in other children, and folic acid and iron supplementation is common.
- Due to the dangers of coincidental chest infection in these patients, prophylactic antibiotics may be considered, particularly in the winter months.
- High-calorie feed and nasogastric or gastrostomy feeds may be required.
- Psychosocial support for the entire family is often indicated due to the chronic nature of the disease.

Mechanical circulatory support

Indications

Increasing ventilation or inotrope requirements, or worsening end-organ function despite maximal medical therapy.

Method of support

- ECMO (see p. 148): indicated for relatively short-term runs (up to 2–3 weeks), for emergency use, or when recovery is thought likely (for instance, with a robust diagnosis of viral myocarditis).
- Ventricular assist device: there is now consensus that ventricular assist device support is associated with a better outcome than ECMO in children bridged to transplantation and should be considered preferable in cases where recovery is thought unlikely within the period of ECMO feasibility.

Risks

- Thrombotic complications are more common than bleeding, and careful attention to optimize anticoagulation is required. Current rates of stroke range from 20% to 48% and significant bleeding 20–59%.
- Anticoagulation is usually a combination of heparin, aspirin, and clopidogrel in small children and warfarin in older.
- Direct thrombin inhibition (bivalirudin) is showing improved outcomes.
- An emerging issue with increasing experience of support of the failing LV is the development of *right heart failure*. Early and late RV impairment poses significant risk and occurs in as many as 25% of patients during long-term support.

Cardiac transplantation

Heart transplantation remains the only long-term viable option for children with end-stage heart failure. Median graft survival is between 15 and 20 years. Transplantation comes at a price, however, of daily immunosuppressants (and other drugs), regular hospital visits, and the risk of important complications, including infection, renal failure, and post-transplant malignancy. Over time, accelerated coronary artery vasculopathy limits the longevity of the transplanted heart.

With donor availability severely limited, transplant programmes must list patients for transplantation only after consideration of many factors, including alternative surgical strategies, likely progression of disease, and systemic comorbidities.

Indications
- Two main groups: (1) cardiomyopathy and (2) CHD.
- The proportion of patients being transplanted for CHD falls with age, with over half of infant recipients being born with CHD compared to less than one-quarter of teenagers.

Contraindications
Cardiovascular
- Anatomical: e.g. severely hypoplastic PAs and PV stenosis, which may require combined heart–lung transplantation.
- Physiological: high PVR (risk of early right heart failure in a donor graft). Pre-listing measurement is advisable if raised PVR is likely.

Comorbidities
- Potential recurrence of a previous malignancy.
- Prognosis of chronic conditions, such as muscular dystrophies and degenerative metabolic conditions.

Psychosocial and learning difficulties
- The ability to cooperate with post-transplant management strategies, particularly medicine compliance, must be considered.

Donor selection
- Donors must be matched with recipients based on size and blood group.
- Blood group compatibility follows that of blood transfusion. However, in young children with immature immune systems, it is sometimes possible to transplant across ABO type, the so-called ABO-incompatible heart transplant. Suitability for this can be assessed by measurement of ABO antibodies prior to transplantation.
- Donor size is mainly based on weight for paediatric recipients (as opposed to height in adult transplantation).
- Overall, in the UK, only 30% of hearts from donors are suitable. Lack of donors means that ~25% of patients listed for transplant will die while waiting for an organ.

Post-transplant management

Immunosuppression

- Immunosuppression is the backbone to a successful outcome post-transplant (Table 11.3).
- The risk of rejection is greatest in the immediate postoperative phase, with hyperacute rejection a potentially devastating event.

Induction immunosuppression

- Around 2/3 of paediatric heart transplant programmes use antilymphocyte induction: antithymocyte globulin (ATG), or specific interleukin-2 antagonists (e.g. basiliximab).

Maintenance immunosuppression

- Tacrolimus (a calcineurin inhibitor) has largely superseded ciclosporin as primary immunosuppression due to better efficacy. In a minority of patients, worsening renal function will preclude further use of tacrolimus, leading to substitution with an mTOR inhibitor (everolimus, sirolimus). In addition, most recipients also receive an antiproliferative agent such as azathioprine or (more commonly) mycophenolate.
- Prednisolone is also commonly used, at least early post-transplantation, when rejection is most likely.
- Over time, the risk of rejection becomes less, and prednisolone is often discontinued. Calcineurin target levels are also lowered after the first year.

Table 11.3 Side effects of common immunosuppressants

Tacrolimus	Renal failure
	Hypertension
	Neurological disturbance (e.g. tremor, headache, seizure at toxic levels)
	Diabetes
	Liver dysfunction
Ciclosporin	Renal failure
	Hypertension
	Hypertrichosis
	Gingival hypertrophy
	Liver dysfunction
Sirolimus	Mouth ulcers
	Hyperlipidaemia
	Pneumonitis
	Anaemia, leucopenia
Mycophenolate	Diarrhoea
	Leucopoenia
	Alopecia
Azathioprine	Bone marrow suppression
	Alopecia
	Liver impairment

Antibiotics

- Bacterial, fungal, and viral infections are common in the immediate postoperative phase when immunosuppression is at its highest, and it is common to give prophylaxis against these for ~3 months.
- Patients who suffer from repeated chest infections may take long-term prophylaxis (e.g. alternate-day azithromycin), particularly during the winter months.

Statins

- Statin use after heart transplantation has been shown to reduce not only coronary allograft vasculopathy, but also rejection and cancer risk.
- They are generally well tolerated, although should be used with caution in infants.

Post-transplant complications

Rejection

- Less than 10% of recipients in the first-year after transplantation.
- Clinical presentation is variable: some will present with non-specific symptoms of abdominal pain and lethargy, others will show signs of significant heart failure, reflecting more severe myocyte injury.
- It is possible for silent acute rejection to occur, which is why many units perform routine endomyocardial biopsy in the first year (when rejection is most likely).
- Non-invasive investigation is useful, but rarely conclusive.
- Reduced voltages on ECG, and diastolic and systolic dysfunction or increasingly pericardial effusion on echocardiography may further raise suspicion, but biopsy remains the gold standard.
- First-line treatment is high dose IV steroids, with antithymocyte globulin (ATG) added for cases with severe haemodynamic compromise.
- It is rare nowadays for an episode in the first year to be fatal, although rejection during this time period is associated with decreased overall survival.
- It is more common in females, re-transplantation, and previous use of ventricular assist device.
- Steroids and IV immunoglobulin are commonly used, but more specific treatments targeted against donor antibody production, such as rituximab, bortezomib, plasmapheresis, and blockage of the complement cascade, are becoming more widespread.

Cardiac allograft vasculopathy

- This is an obliterative microvasculopathy, resulting in intima–medial thickening throughout the coronary vasculature.
- Exacerbating factors include immunological (rejection, infection) and conventional factors (hypertension, smoking, diabetes).
- The diffuse nature of the disease means that coronary intervention via stenting has little impact on clinical outcome, despite often severe stenoses.
- Current figures show ~50% of paediatric patients remain free of the disease at 15 years post-transplantation, although this may represent underdiagnosis due to paucity of adequate surveillance.

- Statin use and sirolimus have been shown to slow progression when initiated early after transplantation, but an effective treatment remains elusive, and cardiac allograft vasculopathy is an important indication for re-transplantation.

Malignancy
- Approximately 1/6 patients will have developed a malignancy by 15 years post-transplantation, with most being affected by post-transplant lymphoproliferative disease, often developing in the lymphoid tissues of the neck, chest, or gut.
- This is almost always Epstein–Barr virus-driven, and should be considered in patients with persistent lymphadenopathy, malaise, or abdominal pain, or derangement of haematological or biochemical parameters.
- More obvious signs such as rectal bleeding or abdominal masses warrant a full work-up including appropriate imaging.

Renal dysfunction
- This is common post-transplantation and is often a combination of poor perfusion pre- and peri-transplantation, and the use of nephrotoxic medications.
- Although it is listed as the cause of death in only ~1% of patients, it is linked to graft loss, and may preclude re-transplantation.
- In severe cases, switching to less nephrotoxic immunosuppressants (e.g. sirolimus) may be indicated.

Hypertension
- At least 1/2 of recipients will be treated for hypertension following transplantation.
- The aetiology combines renal dysfunction, denervation, and drug side effects.
- Treatment is usually with ACEi or calcium channel blockers; beta-blockers are relatively contraindicated due to the risk of profound bradycardia in the denervated heart.

Outcome
- Overall survival following paediatric heart transplantation has improved greatly over the course of the last 20 years.
- The latest international registry figures suggest a median survival of around 15 years, and for those patients alive 1 year post-transplantation, it increases to over 20 years; both figures are predicted to be an underestimate for patients transplanted today.
- Transplantation as an infant or younger child (with an immature immune system) is associated with better outcome.
- Patients transplanted from ECMO have a poorer survival, whereas those stabilized with a period of ventricular assist device support have a similar outlook to those transplanted without support.

Paediatric pulmonary hypertension

Overview

Pulmonary hypertension (PH) is defined haemodynamically as a resting mean pulmonary artery pressure (mPAP) >20 mmHg, beyond the first few months of life. This elevation in mPAP may exist in different physiological forms and in association with numerous medical conditions. It is almost universally associated with significant morbidity and poor survival, due to progressive RV failure.

Physiological types

mPAP is proportional to pulmonary blood flow and PVR but is also dependent on 'downstream' (post-capillary) pulmonary venous or LA pressure. This relationship informs the physiological classification:

- *Elevated PVR*: this is termed pulmonary arterial hypertension (PAH): characterized by progressive luminal narrowing of the PAs. A form of 'pre-capillary' PH.
- *Reduced cross-sectional area of the arteriolar bed*: in conditions of lung hypoplasia (e.g. congenital diaphragmatic hernia), elevated PVR may result from there being fewer arterioles. Also a form of 'pre-capillary' PH.
- *Elevated 'downstream' pressure*: often referred to as 'left heart disease PH'. May occur in patients with pulmonary venous, mitral, or aortic valvar stenosis. A form of 'post-capillary' PH.
- *Increased pulmonary blood flow*: of particular importance in children, the most common example is CHD with a left-to-right shunt lesion.

Many children will have components of more than one physiological type. Differentiating between these is vital when planning the treatment strategy.

Assessment

The goal of assessment is to answer the following questions:

- Does the patient have PH?
- What is the physiological type of PH?
- What is the aetiology?
- How severe is the PH?

This information is used to establish the optimal treatment strategy.

History and examination

- *Symptoms*: dyspnoea, effort intolerance, syncope. *Development of these symptoms without satisfactory explanation should prompt consideration of PH as a cause.*
- *Signs*: accentuated P2, RV heave, hepatomegaly, and elevated jugular venous pressure.

Initial assessment should also include screening for the multitude of conditions PH is associated with, and investigation for important contributory factors in children such as gastro-oesophageal reflux disease ± aspiration and obstructive sleep apnoea. *Treatment of the underlying cause is associated with significant improvements in PH.*

Investigations
- *CXR*: may help differentiate between patients with high pulmonary blood flow (plethora) and those with elevated PVR (oligaemia) as well as identifying those with PH secondary to respiratory disease.
- *ECG*: right axis deviation, RVH (increased amplitude of R wave and S wave in V1 and V6 respectively), QTc may be prolonged. The underlying heart rhythm should be noted.
- *TTE*: the most useful non-invasive test to establish the presence of PH. Systolic PAP is estimated from the tricuspid regurgitation jet velocity, but its absence does not exclude PH. Assessment of the RV should include grading of dilatation, hypertrophy, and function.
- *Cardiac catheterization*: permits direct measurement of PAP, PCWP/LA pressure, and estimation of pulmonary blood flow.
- *Cardiac MRI*: enables assessment of RV function as well as cardiac output and therefore Qp:Qs where shunt lesions are present. Provides useful serial data, but in younger children use may be limited by the need for GA.
- *CT*: characterizes suspected lung pathology and when performed with contrast is helpful in clarifying PV stenosis suspected on echocardiography.

Severity stratification
There is no universally accepted strategy to establish the severity of PH. From the patient's perspective, severity is experienced through functional capacity (assessed using the World Health Organization (WHO) classification). In children, failure to thrive is an indicator of poor prognosis. RV function has shown strong association with prognosis. Interestingly, PAP and PVR are less well correlated with prognosis.

Treatment
Should be preceded by thorough assessment. For most patients treatment is lifelong and will not be curative. In patients with progressive pulmonary vascular disease, treatment goals are to *improve how patients feel and function and to improve survival*.

General measures
- Treatment of underlying causes and contributors such as obstructive sleep apnoea and gastro-oesophageal reflux disease ± aspiration.
- Encouragement to maintain an active lifestyle.
- Avoidance of strenuous exercise, particularly isometric effort in patients with syncope/pre syncope.
- Maintenance of immunization schedules (respiratory syncytial virus prophylaxis recommended).
- Air travel is not contraindicated, and the vast majority of patients will not require supplemental oxygen.

Procedures requiring GA
Consideration must be given to the balance of procedure risk and benefit. It is preferable to carry out procedures in a centre with experienced cardiac anaesthetists. Careful planning and relevant expertise mitigate risk.

Supplemental therapy

Oxygen may be used where there is alveolar hypoxia to counter the effects of hypoxia-mediated vasoconstriction. Diuretics may help to improve symptoms of venous congestion and reduce oedema. Care should be taken to avoid rapid diuresis as this may lead to excessive reduction in RV preload.

Targeted therapy

- *Phosphodiesterase-5 (PDE-5) inhibitors* (sildenafil, tadalafil): PDE-5 is responsible for hydrolysing cGMP (vasodilator). Side effects include dizziness, erections, and systemic hypotension.
- *Endothelin receptor antagonists* (bosentan, macitentan): endothelin drives fibrosis, vascular proliferation, and vasoconstriction (require monthly monitoring of LFTs).
- *Prostacyclin* and its analogues (epoprostenol, treprostinil): potent pulmonary vasodilator with antiproliferative effects (most commonly delivered in inhaled and IV forms).

Mechanical interventions

Considered in patients with advanced disease or disease refractory to therapy. Balloon atrial septostomy (BAS) or the creation of a Pott's shunt (anastomosis between the left PA and descending aorta) provides a 'blow off' to direct blood away from the pulmonary vascular bed and in doing so, relieves RV pressure. Cardiac output is maintained at the expense of normal saturations ('conversion to Eisenmenger physiology').

Bilateral lung transplantation is considered in patients who remain markedly symptomatic despite maximal therapy and who have a poor prognosis. The median survival following lung transplantation for PH is 7 years.

Idiopathic pulmonary arterial hypertension (IPAH)

Idiopathic pulmonary arterial hypertension (IPAH)

IPAH is a form of PAH. It is a progressive disease of the pulmonary vasculature characterized by increased PVR, RV failure, and death. It is a rare condition (UK incidence: 0.5 cases per million children per year, male > female).

Presentation can be throughout childhood, even in infancy. The commonest misdiagnosis is of asthma.

Familial IPAH (majority: *BMPR2* mutations) accounts for 6% of cases and shows genetic anticipation.

Adverse prognostic markers

- Decline in functional capacity (WHO classification).
- Decline in 6-minute walk distance (6MWD).
- RV failure.

Median untreated survival is <1 year and with treatment is 7 years.

Pulmonary arterial hypertension associated with congenital heart disease

Classification

Several types are recognized clinically:

- Eisenmenger syndrome (ES).
- Systemic-to-pulmonary shunts with elevated PVR (shunt cannot be closed without high risks).
- Small cardiac lesions which are not causative but incidental.
- High PVR after corrective cardiac surgery: 2/3 cases of PH associated with CHD occur following corrective surgery and this form carries a poor prognosis.
- Groups require separate management strategies and respond differently to treatment.

Management

Prevention of PAH may be achieved by timely correction of the shunt lesion (prior to development of pulmonary vascular disease).

There are limited data available to define safe thresholds for surgical repair of the underlying shunt lesion; however, a threshold value of indexed PVR <6 Wood units.m^2 reflects consensus opinion. The role of pulmonary vasodilator therapy in these patients remains controversial.

Eisenmenger syndrome (ES)

ES is a form of PAH associated with CHD. It includes all intra- and extracardiac defects beginning as non-restrictive left-to-right shunts and progressing as follows:

- Initial high pulmonary blood flow and left-to-right shunt leading to shear stress/circumferential stretch.
- Endothelial dysfunction and pulmonary vascular remodelling leading to increased PVR.
- Shunt reversal (pulmonary to systemic/right to left) leading to cyanosis.

As the pulmonary vasculature progressively narrows, flow is reduced, and the predominant issue becomes elevated PVR. At this point surgical intervention to repair the lesion is contraindicated: PVR > SVR, shunt reversal maintains cardiac output (at the expense of saturations). Adults with ES have a better survival than those with IPAH.

Around 10% of patients with CHD develop ES. The risk varies according to the underlying defect; children with VSD or AVSD are up to five times more likely to develop PAH than those with an ASD.

Incidence is influenced by rates of detection of CHD and access to surgery.

Presentation

Characterized by severely impaired effort tolerance and multiorgan involvement.

Signs

Cyanosis with clubbing (patients with ES secondary to PDA may have differential cyanosis: SaO_2 upper limb > SaO_2 lower limb, and clubbing of the toes only), accentuated P2, RV heave, murmur from the underlying shunt may be absent as pressures equalize.

Adverse prognostic markers specific to ES include:

- Arrhythmia
- Rising serum uric acid.

Assessment

- *Bloods*: iron status, FBC, serum uric acid.
  - Iron deficiency is reported in over half of patients with ES, reflecting increased red blood cell turnover. It is associated with reduced exercise capacity and higher mortality independently of the presence of anaemia. Patients require regular monitoring with iron supplementation as indicated.
- *CXR*: proximal PA prominence, oligaemic lung fields.
- *ECG*: right axis deviation, RVH (increased amplitude of R wave and S wave in V1 and V6 respectively). The underlying heart rhythm should be noted.
- *TTE*:
  - Establish presence of PH.
  - Characterize underlying CHD.
  - Serial RV assessment (dilation, hypertrophy, and function).

- *Cardiac catheterization*: the risk in children with established ES frequently outweighs potential benefit, meaning it is usually limited to cases of diagnostic uncertainty.
- *Cardiac MRI*: assessment of RV function provides useful serial and prognostic data.

Treatment

General measures
- Active lifestyle.
- Adequate hydration.
- Endocarditis prophylaxis.
- Low threshold for antibiotic treatment of suspected bacterial infections.

Supportive therapy
- Oral anticoagulant treatment is controversial: a high incidence of PA thrombus and stroke is reported, as is an increased risk of haemorrhage and haemoptysis.
- No evidence to support the use of supplemental oxygen in patients without alveolar hypoxia.
- Diuretics may relieve symptoms of venous congestion due to RV failure; care should be taken to avoid dehydration.

Targeted therapy
- There remains uncertainty around the long-term effects of selective pulmonary vasodilators with published data on morbidity and mortality lacking.

Transplantation
- Patients with ES due to simple shunts have been treated with isolated bilateral lung transplantation and repair of the cardiac defect. Treatment is limited by donor availability.

Persistent pulmonary hypertension of the newborn (PPHN)

Successful adaptation to extrauterine life involves a rapid increase in pulmonary blood flow to establish the lung as the site of gas exchange. PPHN is failure of the normal circulatory transition and occurs in 1–2 per 1000 live births. It is most common in term/post-term infants.

Predisposing factors include birth asphyxia, parenchymal lung disease (meconium aspiration syndrome, respiratory distress syndrome, pneumonia, lung hypoplasia due to, e.g. oligohydramnios or congenital diaphragmatic hernia), and maternal non-steroidal anti-inflammatory drug (NSAID)/selective serotonin reuptake inhibitor use.

Important differential diagnosis: cyanotic CHD, particularly obstructed TAPVD (suspect if cardiomegaly, weak pulses, pulmonary oedema).

PPHN usually manifests within 12 hours of life. Presenting features include cyanosis and tachypnoea. In the presence of an arterial duct there may be differential cyanosis (lower limb sats < upper limb >10%). Severity ranges from mild hypoxaemia only, to severe hypoxia with cardiovascular instability.

Physiology

High PVR leads to right-to-left blood flow across the arterial duct, there may also be right-to-left flow across a PFO.

Management

The goal is to reverse hypoxia, improve blood flow to the lungs, and minimize end-organ injury. Echocardiography is useful to rule out important cyanotic CHD, estimate the PA systolic pressure, and define the presence and magnitude of shunts.

- Supportive care (optimize temperature and nutrition, sedation and analgesia, minimal handling, and oxygen).
- Intubation and mechanical ventilation ('gentle' strategy but with appropriate pressures to maintain good lung inflation).
- Inhaled nitric oxide (potent pulmonary vasodilator).
- Haemodynamic support (volume, inotropes).
- ECMO in patients who fail conventional management.

Other causes of pulmonary hypertension in children

Left heart disease PH

- Elevated downstream pressure (beyond the PAs) contributes to elevated PAP by passive transmission through the pulmonary vascular bed.
- In some children secondary changes in the pulmonary arterial tree may result in elevated PVR.
- An important cause in children is *pulmonary vein stenosis, most often seen following preterm birth or previous cardiac surgery* (consider further evaluation with cardiac CT).
- Other causes include mitral valve stenosis, and LV systolic or diastolic dysfunction.

PH associated with respiratory disease: bronchopulmonary dysplasia (BPD)

- BPD accounts for 15% of the paediatric PH population.
- There is currently no standardized screening protocol for PH in BPD patients.
- The pathogenesis of PH in BPD patients is complex and includes interaction between genetic, epigenetic, environmental, and acquired factors such as hyperoxia, hypoxia, infection, and inflammation.
- Management involves optimizing growth and development of lungs, and treatment of contributory factors.
- The role of pulmonary vasodilator therapy in this group of patients is controversial due to a paucity of published data.
- For patients with BPD PH who survive beyond 6 months, resolution of PH is likely.

Multisystem disorders

Rheumatic fever

- *Acute rheumatic fever* (ARF) represents an autoimmune reaction to bacterial infection (usually pharyngitis) caused by group A *Streptococcus* (GAS), predominantly seen in school-age children.
- *Rheumatic carditis* is the acute inflammatory reaction of cardiac tissues, predominantly the mitral and aortic valves, associated with ARF.
- *Rheumatic heart disease* (RHD) is the long-term cardiac manifestation of severe or recurrent ARF causing recurrent carditis leading primarily to heart valve disease, most commonly seen in adults over the age of 30 (although may present early).

ARF can lead to severe multisystem inflammation and acute heart failure; treatment is aimed at eradication of bacterial infection and medical support of acute inflammation and heart failure.

Primary prevention of the initial episode of ARF is challenging but secondary prevention of recurrent rheumatic fever and resultant RHD is the main focus of treatment.

Incidence

ARF and RHD are now uncommon in Europe and North America. ARF remains endemic in certain regions including sub-Saharan Africa, South Asia, and Australasia (predominantly in indigenous populations). ARF and RHD are the leading causes of cardiovascular death in the first five decades of life in these countries.

Diagnosis

- There is no single diagnostic test for ARF.
- A clinical syndrome of ARF is defined using the Jones criteria (updated 2015). To confirm the diagnosis of a first episode of rheumatic fever: either two major criteria or one major and two minor criteria (Table 13.1), plus laboratory evidence of a recent GAS throat infection.

Clinical findings

ARF should be suspected in any child with persistent fever, a new heart murmur, and/or signs of acute heart failure. May also be associated multisystem involvement with a transient polyarthritis, characteristic skin lesions, or neurological findings. New apical pansystolic murmur consistent with mitral regurgitation, minor ECG changes including first-degree heart block, and any signs of acute heart failure suggest acute rheumatic carditis.

Table 13.1 Abbreviated Jones criteria for diagnosis of rheumatic fever

Major	Minor
Carditis	Fever
Arthritis	Arthralgia
Chorea	Raised erythrocyte sedimentation rate/C-reactive protein
Erythema marginatum	Prolonged PR interval
Subcutaneous nodules	

Echocardiography may show evidence of valve inflammation, primarily mitral regurgitation, and/or aortic incompetence. Cardiac function can be normal, depressed, or commonly hyperdynamic due to valvar regurgitation and fever. Pericardial effusions may be present.

Treatment

Primary prevention of ARF requires adequate and appropriate treatment for GAS pharyngitis. This is reliant on symptom severity prompting medical review, accessibility to healthcare, plus correct diagnosis and completion of appropriate treatment regimen. In endemic areas, many GAS infections do not reach this threshold and therefore are not treated, thus impacting the effectiveness of primary prevention.

Secondary prevention is a major focus worldwide to minimize the morbidity and mortality associated with ARF/RHD. The aim is to prevent GAS reinfection and thus prevent recurrent ARF. GAS infections may be asymptomatic and in addition, recurrent rheumatic fever may occur even if a symptomatic GAS infection has been treated adequately. Once a child or young adult has been diagnosed with ARF, a treatment course of penicillin aims to treat acute infection and eradicate pharyngeal carriage of the bacterium.

Subsequent long-term (until age 21 years) penicillin prophylaxis is then initiated to prevent GAS reinfection and hence reduce the risk of recurrent ARF. Programmes using regular (every 3–4 weeks) deep intramuscular penicillin in high-risk populations and in endemic regions have been most successful.

* For children with ARF, inpatient care, strict bed rest, and anti-failure medications are recommended. Heart failure should be managed using established protocols including diuretics and ACEi.
* Anti-inflammatory medications including corticosteroids are commonly used but clear evidence for benefit from anti-inflammatories and steroids is lacking.

Rheumatic heart disease

RHD is the chronic evolution of severe or recurrent ARF. The commonest chronic lesion is mitral stenosis or mixed mitral valve disease with both mitral regurgitation and stenosis, due to thickened chordae and fibrotic valve tissue leading to restricted opening and closing of valve apparatus. Established fibrotic mitral stenosis takes time to develop and children may present primarily with mitral regurgitation.

Echocardiography

* The mitral valve leaflets are thickened, sometimes calcified, and have reduced excursion.
* Doppler assessment of valve gradients and 2D assessment of valve orifice area is essential in follow-up.
* 3D echocardiography adds further definition.
* Similarly, aortic valve stenosis, but more commonly aortic incompetence is the presenting feature.
* Aortic regurgitation usually coexists with mitral valve disease rather than as isolated mixed aortic valve disease.

Management
- Medical management is the mainstay of treatment.
- Catheter intervention for mitral stenosis is available, with cardiac surgery reserved for refractory heart failure due to valvar regurgitation.

Kawasaki disease (KD)

Kawasaki disease (KD)

KD is a systemic vasculitis that is now the commonest cause of acquired heart disease in children in developed countries. Cardiac involvement: coronary dilatation ± aneurysm formation in up to 25% of untreated patients, myocarditis/pancarditis, and rare instances of cardiovascular shock syndromes.

Aetiology and epidemiology

Multifactorial causality including genetic disposition, environmental, and potentially infective triggers. KD predominantly affects infants and pre-school-age children. Seasonal influence with higher incidence in winter and spring in northern hemisphere countries.

Genetic and environmental influences are also likely. KD was first described in Japan, with prevalence there still higher than elsewhere, but KD is also more prevalent in children of Japanese ancestry who live elsewhere (e.g. Hawaii).

Diagnosis

There is no specific diagnostic test for KD; diagnosis is based on clinical criteria. For the diagnosis of 'complete' or 'classical' KD, the child must have fever for >4 days with four out of five of the features shown in Table 13.2. Fever may be of shorter duration if all five criteria are present. KD may be diagnosed with fewer than four of the features if coronary artery abnormalities are detected.

Incomplete/atypical KD

The diagnosis of KD should be considered in any child with a prolonged febrile exanthematous illness who also has evidence of inflammation. Children with incomplete (also known as atypical) KD do not fulfil all diagnostic criteria but are still at risk of cardiac involvement, especially high-risk groups such as infants.

Cardiac findings

Coronary artery involvement

- Coronary artery dilatation is most common 1–2 weeks after fever.
- In a minority, coronary artery aneurysms will then occur.

Table 13.2 Diagnostic testing for KD

1. **Oral changes**	Red/cracked lips, strawberry tongue, oropharyngeal mucosal erythema
2. **Eye changes**	Bilateral, bulbar, non-exudative conjunctivitis
3. **Rash**	Maculopapular, diffuse erythroderma or erythema multiforme
4. **Peripheral changes**	Hand/foot oedema (acute) Desquamation (subacute)
5. **Lymphadenopathy**	Cervical, >1.5 cm commonly unilateral

- If mild (Z score <+2.5) often returns to baseline after inflammation settles.
- Early diagnosis, with early use of intravenous immunoglobulin (IVIG) has reduced the incidence of subsequent coronary aneurysms from 25% in untreated cases to <5% after treatment.

Widespread pancarditis
- Pericardial effusion (usually small).
- Valvar regurgitation (usually mitral).
- ECG changes including:
  - Prolongation of PR interval
  - Non-specific voltage changes
  - Ventricular repolarization changes.

Systolic myocardial function may be impaired—best assessed using advanced echocardiographic techniques (speckle-tracking echocardiography and tissue Doppler imaging).

Treatment

Treatment should be initiated as soon as KD is diagnosed—irrespective of complete or incomplete:
- IVIG is the mainstay of treatment as a continuous infusion over 6–12 hours.
- High-dose aspirin in four divided doses should also be given until fever has settled for 48 hours, clinical improvement has occurred, and C-reactive protein level decreasing.
- Following this, low-dose (antiplatelet dose) aspirin is indicated for all children with KD for a minimum of 6 weeks.
- Coronary aneurysms may require anticoagulation:
  - In giant aneurysms (Z score >+10) formal oral anticoagulation is recommended after heparinization.
  - In small- (Z score +2.5 to +5) to medium-size aneurysms (z score +5 to +10), an individualized approach can be adopted using aspirin, clopidogrel, low-molecular-weight heparin, or oral anticoagulants according to individual risk assessment, age, and other comorbidities.

Treatment of severe KD
Treatment may need to be escalated if there are signs of severe disease:
- IVIG resistance, i.e. ongoing fever/inflammation/clinical signs.
- Features of haemophagocytic lymphohistiocytosis.
- Shock.
- Under 1 year of age.
- Presentation with coronary and/or peripheral aneurysms.

Treatment escalations should be individualized and monitored by relevant subspecialities (Immunology/infectious diseases, rheumatology, general paediatrics, and cardiology).
  Options include:
- Repeat IVIG infusion
- Corticosteroids
- Tumour necrosis factor (TNF)-alpha blockade (e.g. infliximab).
- In refractory cases other biologics and/or immunosuppressive agents (e.g ciclosporin) may be considered by subspecialty teams

Follow-up

All children with KD should have structured MDT follow-up.

Blood tests (FBC, CRP, LFTs, U&E) are monitored until they have returned to normal baseline. If ongoing concern of macrophage activation syndrome, then ferritin and fibrinogen should also be monitored.

At diagnosis
- Monitor patients daily (clinical observations, inflammatory markers) until afebrile.
- Baseline TTE at diagnosis is recommended.
- In cases with signs of carditis or coronary dilatation, frequent TTE until changes have stabilized.
- Once afebrile, high-dose aspirin is changed to low-dose thromboprophylaxis.
- Low-dose aspirin thromboprophylaxis as single daily dose should be continued at least until after the 6–8-week TTE and clinical review.

At 2 weeks after onset of fever

Clinical and echocardiographic review, as this is the time for maximum coronary involvement.
- If coronary involvement has worsened since diagnosis, more detailed imaging with ECG-gated coronary CT is undertaken to establish baseline measurements.
- For those with ongoing cardiac change, inpatient MDT review will look for evidence of persistent or recurrent inflammation and manage accordingly.
- Cardiac monitoring with ECG and TTE should be planned once or twice per week until coronary changes stabilize.

At 6 weeks after onset of fever

If TTE has been initially and subsequently normal, aspirin can stop at 6 weeks.

At 6 months and at 12 months

For those with no ongoing inflammation and with normal or stable TTE, interval review should be scheduled for 6 months and if normal, again at 12 months. If all TTEs have been normal throughout, children can be discharged from further KD follow-up at 12 months. For those with coronary dilatation or aneurysms, indefinite follow-up is required.

Longer-term considerations

Established coronary aneurysms put an individual at risk of future acute cardiac events, including ischaemic acute coronary syndromes (ACS). At-risk children and young people should have an individualized management plan agreed in advance and updated regularly.

Patient-specific passports serve to alert emergency services to redirect children and young adults with an ACS to a designated centre able to offer time-critical paediatric cardiology assessment, coronary investigations, and acute coronary intervention on the same site.

Although ACS events are rare, a prompt multilevel response is needed. Therefore, a regional approach with a single paediatric ACS centre co-located with an adult heart attack centre is encouraged.

Infectious endocarditis (IE)

IE is infection of the endocardial surface of the heart. The intracardiac lesions can cause valvar insufficiency, which may lead to intractable congestive heart failure, and myocardial abscesses.

Aetiology

- Any type of structural heart disease can predispose to IE, including CHD and acquired lesions such as RHD.
- Other risk factors include prosthetic heart valves and implanted devices.
- *Staphylococcus aureus* followed by streptococci of the viridans group and coagulase-negative staphylococci are the three most common organisms responsible for IE.
- HACEK group of microorganisms (*Haemophilus* spp., *Aggregatibacter* (previously *Actinobacillus*) *actinomycetemcomitans*, *Cardiobacterium hominis*, *Eikenella corodens*, and *Kingella kingae*) and fungi are seen less frequently.

Clinical presentation

- Fever occurs in 97% of patients.
- Malaise and fatigue in 90%.
- A new or changing heart murmur.
- Weight loss.
- Cough.
- Vascular phenomena or immunological phenomena as outlined in the modified Duke's criteria, shown below.
- Other features may include night sweats, rigors, anaemia, or splenomegaly.

The modified Duke's criteria are used for the diagnosis of IE:

Major criteria

1. Two positive blood cultures (drawn >12 hours apart).
2. Evidence of endocardial involvement on echocardiogram (oscillating mass, abscess, dehiscence of prosthetic valve, new valvar regurgitation).

Minor criteria

1. Predisposing condition (structural cardiac lesion or IV drug use).
2. Fever >38°C.
3. Vascular phenomena (arterial emboli, septic pulmonary infarcts, infectious aneurysm, intracranial haemorrhage, conjunctival haemorrhage, or Janeway lesions).
4. Immunological phenomena (Osler nodes, Roth spots, rheumatoid factor on blood test).
5. Microbiological or serological evidence that does not meet a major criterion.

Definite diagnosis of IE

- Two major criteria, *or*
- One major and three minor criteria, *or*
- Five minor criteria.

Possible diagnosis of IE
- One major and one minor criterion, *or*
- Three minor criteria.

Management

Medical management
- Input from infectious diseases and microbiology teams should always be considered.
- The antibiotic treatment should be tailored to each patient according to strain resistance.
- It is likely that a prolonged course of IV antibiotics will be required.

Surgical management
Surgery may be required for tissue debridement, repair of intracardiac lesions, or prosthetic material removal/replacement.

Avoidance of infectious endocarditis

Patients with CHD should maintain good oral hygiene and avoid and body piercings. Guidance for antibiotic prophylaxis for dental procedures in at-risk patients varies between countries. In the UK, the National Institute for Health and Care Excellence does not recommend antibiotic prophylaxis to cover such procedures. Other groups, such as the European Society of Cardiology, continue to recommend antibiotic prophylaxis for high-risk groups (e.g. prosthetic valves). Unit/region-specific guidance should be consulted.

Pericardial disease

Pericardial disease is a relatively common cause of chest pain in children. The term includes both pericardial inflammation (pericarditis) and fluid accumulation in the pericardial space (pericardial effusion). There is considerable overlap in aetiology, presentation, and management between the two groups.

Aetiology

The most common causes of pericardial disease in children are:

Infectious causes
- *Viral* (common): enteroviruses, herpesviruses, adenoviruses, parvovirus B19.
- *Bacterial* (rare): *Pneumococcus* spp., *Meningococcus* spp., *Gonococcus* spp., *Streptococcus* spp., *Staphylococcus* spp., *Mycobacterium tuberculosis*.
- *Fungal* (very rare).

Non-infectious causes
- *Autoimmune (common)*: systemic lupus erythematosus, Sjögren syndrome, rheumatoid arthritis, scleroderma, systemic vasculitis syndromes.
- *Neoplastic*: primary tumours (rare), secondary metastatic tumours.
- *Metabolic*: uraemia, myxoedema, anorexia nervosa.
- *Indirect injury* (non-penetrating thoracic injury, radiation injury).
- *Post-pericardiotomy syndrome*: following cardiac surgery, most commonly surgical repair of ASD.
- *Drug related (rare)*: antineoplastic drugs, granulocyte-macrophage colony-stimulating factor (GM-CSF), anti-TNF agents.
- *Other (uncommon)*: congenital partial and complete absence of the pericardium, amyloidosis, aortic dissection, PAH, and chronic heart failure.

Clinical features

Acute pericarditis
- Chest pain (often central/left-sided, sharp, worse on inspiration, and on lying flat).
- Fever (often low grade).
- Pericardial rub on auscultation ('walking on snow').
- ECG: widespread saddle-shaped ST elevation or PR depression.
- Elevated inflammatory markers (C-reactive protein, erythrocyte sedimentation rate, and white blood cell count).
- Evidence of pericardial thickening on CT or MRI.
- *Constrictive pericarditis* is rare in children but presents with the above plus evidence of right heart failure.

Pericardial effusion
- Symptoms depend on the speed of pericardial fluid accumulation (slowly accumulating fluid may be well tolerated).
- Dyspnoea on exertion.
- Orthopnoea.
- Chest pain.
- Muffled heart sounds.

The following are signs of *cardiac tamponade* (compression of the heart by the accumulating effusion, a life-threatening cardiac emergency):

- Tachycardia.
- Hypotension.
- Pulsus paradoxus.
- Raised jugular venous pressure.

Management

Medical

- NSAIDs are the mainstay of medical management and should be used as first-line treatment.
- Second-line options include:
  - Colchicine
  - Corticosteroids
  - Anakinra (anti-IL1 receptor antagonist).

Interventional/surgical

- Cardiac tamponade or worsening pericardial effusion should be drained by needle pericardiocentesis (see p. 169).
- Chronic pericardial effusions are sometimes managed by the creation of a surgical pericardial-pleural window.
- Constrictive pericarditis may require pericardectomy, typically after bacterial or TB infection.

Outcome

The outcome of viral or idiopathic pericarditis (and post-pericardiotomy syndrome) in children is largely very good with conservative management. Other causes may have a more guarded prognosis. Recurrent (multiple episodes separated by a symptom-free window of >4 weeks) or chronic (lasting >3 months) pericarditis can occur, which can be more difficult to treat.

Systemic arterial hypertension

Normal BP ranges in children are influenced by factors such as age, height, and sex, thus a single definition of hypertension (HTN) cannot apply to all children. Furthermore, HTN should not be diagnosed on a single reading. Most authorities base the definition on measurement of elevated systolic and/or diastolic BP on three consecutive readings. HTN is defined as readings above the 95th percentile for age, height, and sex.

How to measure BP

BP should be measured in the right arm with the child at rest, using an appropriately sized cuff. Strictly speaking, elevated oscillometric measurement should be confirmed by auscultatory measurement. Ambulatory BP monitoring is often employed to confirm HTN and provides longer-term monitoring, both day and night, to allow monitoring and observe normal patterns such as night-time dipping of BP.

Normal BP ranges in children are briefly summarized in Table 13.3.

More detailed analysis can be found at https://www.bcm.edu/body complab/BPappZjs/BPvAgeAPPz.html.

Aetiology

If no underlying cause to explain raised BP can be identified, this is termed *essential* or *primary* HTN, and if an underlying cause is identified, this is *secondary* HTN. Other important scenarios include 'white coat HTN' where BP is elevated in a clinic setting but normal otherwise, and 'masked' HTN where clinic BP is normal but ambulatory measures are abnormal.

Essential HTN is strongly linked to obesity, particularly in male adolescents.

Secondary HTN causes include

- Renal disease, e.g. polycystic kidneys, acute kidney injury.
- Cardiac disease, e.g. coarctation of the aorta, mid-aortic syndrome.
- Vascular, e.g. renal artery stenosis, haemolytic uraemic syndrome.
- Tumours, e.g. phaeochromocytoma, neuroblastoma.
- Endocrine, e.g. congenital adrenal hyperplasia, Cushing's disease, hyperthyroidism.
- Genetic, e.g. Liddle syndrome (pseudo-aldosteronism), tuberous sclerosis, neurofibromatosis.

Table 13.3 Approximate normal BP ranges at a variety of different ages

Age	Systolic BP (mmHg)	Diastolic BP (mmHg)
12 hours	50–70	24–45
3 days	60–90	20–60
6 months	87–105	53–66
2 years	95–105	53–66
7 years	97–112	57–71
15 years	112–128	68–80

- Medications, e.g. corticosteroids.
- Obesity.
- Miscellaneous, e.g. obstructive sleep apnoea, prematurity.

Approach to diagnosis

History

- Symptoms are present in a minority of cases.
- Family history of HTN.
- Preterm delivery.
- Symptoms of upper airways obstruction.

Physical examination

- Femoral pulses.
- Tachycardia can be due to medical setting or underlying endocrine cause (e.g. phaeochromocytoma).
- Signs of Cushing's disease (e.g. striae, acanthosis nigricans).
- Thyroid examination for enlargement.
- Ophthalmic examination for severe HTN for papilloedema and retinal changes.

Investigations

- Blood: urea, creatinine, electrolytes, lipids, liver function.
- Urinalysis (blood, protein).
- Renal ultrasound scan (including renal artery Doppler).
- TTE (exclude coarctation and assess for LV hypertrophy).
- Depending on history/examination, other investigations may include:
  - Plasma renin activity
  - Thyroid function
  - Serum cortisol/adrenocorticotropic hormone
  - Serum metanephrines
  - Dimercaptosuccinic acid (DMSA) scan
  - Micturating cystourethrogram (MCUG)
  - Sleep study
  - MRI/CT of aortic arch/renal arteries.

Treatment

- Weight loss and exercise/dietary input for essential HTN, particularly if overweight.
- Underlying condition leading to HTN should be treated for secondary HTN.
- Drug therapy can be considered depending on cause (consider input from paediatric nephrologist):
  - ACEi.
  - Angiotensin receptor blocker.
  - Calcium channel blocker.
  - Beta-blocker.
  - Diuretics.

Stroke

A full description of the aetiology and management of children presenting with stroke is beyond the scope of this handbook—the focus of this section is to outline risk groups for stroke, including those children with a normal heart structure and those with underlying cardiac disease.

Types of stroke

Strokes may be broadly subdivided into:
- Haemorrhagic stroke
- Arterial ischaemic stroke, usually caused by thromboembolism.

It is important to recognize that haemorrhage into an ischaemic area of the brain may occur.

The assessment and management of paediatric stroke is typically led by paediatric neurologists. Paediatric cardiologists often become involved to help define a source of embolism. Underlying CHD is a recognized risk factor for stroke.

Cardiac disease and stroke risk

The following all increase the risk of stroke:
- Reduced cardiac function:
  - Cardiomyopathy/myocarditis.
  - Persistent arrhythmia causing poor function.
- Cardiac arrhythmia: atrial flutter/SVT/PJRT/VT.
- Single-ventricle physiology:
  - Thrombus within atriums/ventricles/blind-ending vessels.
  - Paradoxical embolism from Fontan pathway through fenestration.
- Unoperated lesions: TGA.
- Infective: vegetations (IE).
- Cardiac masses: atrial myxoma (rare in children).
- Iatrogenic:
  - Post CPB.
  - Septostomy.
  - Placement of devices (e.g. ASD occluder).
  - Indwelling venous catheters via paradoxical embolism.

Paradoxical embolism

- This is the embolism of a thrombus from a systemic vein across an intracardiac shunt to the left side of the heart, and then the brain, causing a stroke.
- This might include right-to-left shunting across a VSD (e.g. ES), or at atrial level across a PFO or ASD.
- In the neonatal period the foramen ovale is normally patent, so identification of PFO does not usually assist (unless thrombus is visualized in either atrium).
- Investigation of systemic veins may help in identification of the source of the embolism.
- Later in life, paradoxical embolism is also considered a potential cause of stroke.

- TTE may show an atrial communication on colour flow Doppler, but the absence of such on TTE or TOE does not exclude the possibility of paradoxical embolism.

Neurological investigations

These should be guided by neurological input, generally including brain CT and/or MRI/magnetic resonance angiogram to confirm embolic stroke and differentiate from other causes.

Cardiac investigations for embolic stroke

Echocardiography

- To assess cardiac structure and function as well as embolic source.
- TTE may yield excellent images in young children and for near-field structures (e.g. ventricular apices).
- TOE has better image quality, particularly in older children/adolescents and is superior for imaging of regions such as atrial appendages and atrial septum.

Saline contrast echocardiography

- If paradoxical embolism is being considered, injection of 5–10 mL of agitated saline on release of the Valsalva manoeuvre permits visualization of right-to-left flow of bubbles from right heart to left heart, confirming potential for right-to-left shunt.
- May be done by TTE/TOE in awake or anaesthetized patient.
- Valsalva under anaesthesia by maintaining 20 cmH$_2$O of positive end-expiratory pressure, then release.

ECG/Holter monitoring

- To exclude occult arrhythmia.

Transition and adult congenital heart disease

Adolescence and transition

The transition process involves addressing the specific needs of adolescents and young adults as they move towards adult services. The end point is the complete transfer of care. Cardiology services should deliver structured transition and transfer of care to ensure continuity of care and account for the patient's unique needs.

Considerations include the following:

- *A change of team*: potentially away from doctors, nurses, and allied health professionals that a patient has known all their life.
- *A shift in responsibility*: during the transition process, patients will become increasingly responsible for their own ongoing care and attendance of hospital appointments. While family are generally still involved, their role becomes more marginal, and parents may require assistance with this.
- *Knowledge and empowerment*: ensuring that patients have a solid understanding of their condition, and its implications, is crucial for their adherence to follow-up and care in adult life.

The process of transition should be individualized, taking the physical, psychological, and emotional development of the patient into consideration. Usually, it begins around 12 years of age with transfer at 16–19 years of age.

Transition timeline

The transition process should start with

- Introduction of the concept and importance of transition and need for ongoing follow-up
- Explanation of what to expect (brief outline of transition process)
- Introducing the transition team and their contact (transition cardiac clinical nurse specialist (CNS), transition administration team).

Building on this with

- Patient education material (lifestyle, disease specific, websites, patient associations)
- Development of a personalized plan: face-to-face clinic, virtual clinic, telephone clinic, and/or seminars
- Formal transition clinics with transition cardiac CNS (face-to-face, virtual, or telephone)
- Complex patients (anatomically complex/those with comorbidities/advanced heart failure/haemodynamically significant lesions) should have a *medical transition* clinic with the paediatric and ACHD consultants, and respective CNSs, in addition to the above.
- Seminars to meet the ACHD team, provide a tour of ACHD facilities, opportunity to meet other young CHD patients and families/carers. These should include sessions without the family, to allow young adults the freedom to ask questions and raise concerns that they may not in the presence of a family member.

15–16 years of age

- Ensure medical transition clinics/contacts have happened, education process is complete, and management plan has been set.
- Offer repeat appointments if necessary.

16–18 years of age
- First ACHD (transfer) clinic: ACHD consultants take over care from paediatric consultants.

18–21 years of age
- Ongoing support from transition team as required.

Lifestyle and exercise

Increasing numbers of children with CHD are surviving into adulthood. As this population ages, they encounter the same cardiovascular risk factors (hypercholesterolaemia, diabetes, hypertension, obesity, and smoking) as the general population.

- 80% of ACHD patients have at least one cardiovascular risk factor, whereas only 20% have a fully heart-healthy lifestyle.
- 30% of ACHD patients are overweight and 10% obese. This is slightly less than the general population, but with a trend that shows a steady increase.

Achieving a healthy lifestyle should be one of the main goals of patient education, ideally starting in adolescence. Clinical physiologists and counselling can play a vital role in achieving lifestyle change, but some patients may also require motivational therapy, delivered by a trained professional.

Lifestyle education includes the followings topics:

Exercise

- Benefits: improvements in skeletal muscle function, vascular health, immune system function, obesity prevention, control of lipid levels, and glucose tolerance as well as complex psychological, cognitive, and social function.
- Benefits accrue with activities of at least moderate intensity (60–70% of target HR).

Exercise recommendations, including type and intensity of exercise, should be individualized, and discussed regularly with ACHD patients.

Many ACHD patients will have a reduced exercise capacity and low exercise self-efficacy. Older age and muscle endurance are both associated with low exercise self-efficacy.

Assessment

- Begins with evaluation of overall fitness and level of exercise tolerance (history ± objective assessment with CPET) to risk stratify and benchmark current levels of fitness.
- Exercise risk factors include arrhythmias, ventricular dysfunction, aortopathy, coronary anomalies, and elevated pulmonary vascular resistance.

Recommendations

Current guidelines recommend the following physical activity:

- Muscle-strengthening activities ≥2 days per week and accumulate 75 minutes of vigorous or 150 minutes of moderate activity per week, with each activity session lasting ≥10 minutes.
- Patients with significant *ventricular dysfunction* can enjoy a wide range of recreational sport and physical activity opportunities, while limiting their involvement in competitive sport.
- Patients with *aortic dilatation* are at increased risk of aortic dissection and should limit activity intensity. Activities of moderate intensity are generally safe.
- Patients with *syncope* should avoid activities with a risk of injury such as horse riding, gymnastics, rock climbing, or scuba diving.

- Patients taking *anticoagulant medications* and with *implantable cardiac devices* should avoid activities in which body impact is an intentional aspect of the sport, such as rugby, combative martial arts, boxing, and ice hockey.
- Patients with *arrhythmia* should follow the recommendations of the Heart Rhythm Society.

Nutrition

A healthy diet includes appropriate caloric intake but also provides quality and nutrients. Patients should be provided with information around refined sugars, sources of protein, type of fats, vitamin and fibre intake, the role of salt, and processed food.

Excessive caloric intake leads to obesity which predisposes to metabolic, mechanical, and psychological comorbidities (e.g. diabetes, hypertension, coronary artery disease, stroke, heart failure, kidney disease, skin infection, sleep apnoea, asthma, depression, anxiety, and low self-esteem). Obesity also causes changes in inflammatory cytokines, which cause a patient to be prothrombotic, an effect that becomes particularly dangerous in patients with arrhythmias, Fontan circulation, cyanosis, or prothrombotic states. The support of a dietician may be required to achieve the desired goal.

Smoking

Smoking remains a leading cause of death in the UK, increasing the risk of vascular diseases, malignancy, and lung damage. Passive smoking poses the same risks but at lower rate. Patients with CHD are at higher risk and so should avoid smoking.

Alcohol

Even in low amounts, alcohol is a known trigger for arrhythmia. In patients using anticoagulants, alcohol may increase bleeding risk. Patients should be aware of such risks and limit consumption to 1–2 units per day.

Recreational drug use

IV drug abuse adds a further 2–5% risk of developing IE.

Education and employability

- ACHD patients should have access to learning opportunities and be encouraged to achieve their goals. Hospital appointments and cardiac procedures can impact school attendance and exam performance.
- A proportion of patients may present with a broad range of learning difficulties, which can be part of a coexisting genetic condition but may also occur as a consequence of neurological injury at the time of surgery. Recognizing their difficulties is key in promptly offering support and obtaining an Education Health and Care Plan (EHCP).
- When looking for a job, factors that need to be taken into account are patients' physical limitation and the job's demand so that a health–life–work balance can be achieved.

Dental hygiene and endocarditis prophylaxis

- IE is a leading cause of morbidity and mortality in patients with CHD.
- The risk of IE is 20–50 times that of the general population (see p. 262).

Contraception and pregnancy

Heart disease is the leading single cause of maternal death in the UK. The risk for ACHD patients relates to their underlying condition.

Ideally, pregnancies should be planned, so that cardiac risk can be assessed for the mother and the fetus.

- Contraceptive counselling is important and should start during transition.
- Before embarking on pregnancy, high-risk lesions need to be identified and treated where possible, risky medications discontinued, and cardiac function and exercise capacity accurately assessed.
- Where pregnancy carries an unacceptably high risk, contraception needs to be highly effective, and either long term or permanent.

Contraception

The cardiovascular safety and contraceptive efficacy of each contraceptive method must be considered in the context of the patient's underlying CHD.

Barrier methods

- User-dependent efficacy (with perfect use 92–98% but typically they have a higher failure rate than other methods).
- Protect against sexually transmitted infections.
- No cardiovascular risk.

Hormonal methods

- Potentially good efficacy (up to 99%) but with typical use there is a 6–9% failure rate.
- The combined pill (oestrogen containing) is not suitable for patients at higher risk of thrombosis, who are cyanosed or are at risk of paradoxical embolism due to the thrombotic effects.
- Progesterone-only methods do not carry a cardiovascular risk and have a high efficacy (99%) in long-acting forms. Efficacy is poorer when taken in oral form.

Implants, intrauterine devices (IUDs), and sterilization

- Guarantee an efficacy of 99%.
- IUDs are long lasting but have associated risk of bacteraemia during insertion and therefore of IE.
- They may cause irregular bleeding.
- Painful menorrhagia is common with traditional copper IUDs.

Emergency contraception

- Ulipristal (anti-progestin) and levonorgestrel (progestin) are used after unprotected sex (and have no cardiac contraindications).
- A copper IUD can also be used as emergency contraception.

Pregnancy

While the majority of CHD patients can tolerate pregnancy well, the pregnancy-related haemodynamic changes can result in complications.

Preconception

Up-to-date assessment and risk stratification (history, examination, ECG, echocardiogram, CPET) additional information (24-hour ECG, MRI, CT, cardiac catheterization may be required). Risks increase with maternal age and disease complexity.

The goal of the assessment is to
- Identify high-risk lesions
- Determine the need for any intervention prior to pregnancy to reduce the risk
- Assess exercise capacity, arrhythmia history, and anticoagulation risk
- Assess medication safety during pregnancy
- Discuss genetic counselling.

A multidisciplinary approach involving an ACHD specialist, maternal fetal medicine specialist, obstetrician, and anaesthetist is essential for those with moderate and severe CHD. Various risk assessment scores are available.

Physiological response to pregnancy
- Blood volume and cardiac output increases by 40%, HR increases by 15–20%.
- During labour, there is a further increase in cardiac output, BP, and finally a shift of blood from the uterus and placenta into the mother's circulation all of which represent a potential risk.

Fetal risk
- Any maternal risk is a risk to the fetus.
- Risk of recurrence of CHD (see p. 194).
- 50% recurrence risk for genetic conditions with autosomal dominant inheritance.
- Involvement of a geneticist may be indicated.
- Drug/alcohol misuse, certain medications, and infections can also have an impact on fetal development.

Specific considerations

Bicuspid aortic valve
- Pregnancy is usually contraindicated if the aorta measures >4.5 cm, if there is severe AS without adequate BP rise during exercise, or severe aortic regurgitation with impairment of LV function.
- New onset or worsening of heart failure as well as arrhythmias are the most common complications during pregnancy.

Repaired tetralogy of Fallot
- Can undergo pregnancy if they are asymptomatic, arrhythmia free, and ventricular volumes and function do not reach threshold for surgery.

Repaired coarctation of the aorta
- The presence of aneurysm or severe re-coarctation generally needs intervention prior to pregnancy.

ccTGA
- Important to assess RV (systemic ventricle) volumes and systolic function and degree of tricuspid valve regurgitation (TTE, cMRI, CPET).

Repaired TGA with Mustard or Senning procedures (atrial switch)
- Can develop RV failure, tricuspid valve regurgitation, baffle occlusion, and/or arrhythmia as result of pregnancy.

- Careful monitoring is required throughout pregnancy and pre-pregnancy assessment of baffle patency, ventricular and tricuspid valve function, and arrhythmias is required.

Single-ventricle circulation (Fontan)
- Pregnancy is possible in these patients with careful pre-conception evaluation, monitoring during pregnancy, and birth planning.
- High risk of miscarriage at about 27%, maternal events (10% excluding death), and low birth weight generally related to lower maternal oxygen levels.

Pulmonary hypertension
- Severe PH is associated with high (up to 50%) maternal mortality and complications such as bleeding, RV failure, PH crisis, thromboembolism, and poor fetal prognosis (intrauterine growth restriction 24%, neonatal death 7%, premature delivery 86%).

Mechanical valves
- Pregnancy is not contraindicated but poses specific challenges—including the anticoagulation regimen, which is still not uniformly agreed on.
- Warfarin is associated with fetal abnormalities and further potential neurological abnormalities during the second and third trimesters.
- Low-molecular-weight heparin is therefore used instead but requires meticulous monitoring (weekly) of anti-Xa-levels; aspirin can be added during the second and third trimesters.
- Patients are, however, at risk of valve thrombosis (5%), higher rate of haemorrhagic complications (23% vs 5%), and higher risk of miscarriage, fetal mortality, and lower birth weight.

Commonly used drugs in paediatric cardiology

Diuretics

- Act on the kidney via various mechanisms to increase sodium and thus water excretion.
- Less commonly used to treat hypertension, compared to adult practice.

Loop diuretics (e.g. furosemide, bumetanide)

- The most powerful class of diuretics.

Mechanism

- Act on the ascending limb of the loop of Henle, inhibiting sodium reabsorption.

Uses in paediatric cardiology

- Heart failure (see p. 234).
- Post cardiac surgery using CPB.
- Fluid retention (e.g. in protein-losing enteropathy).

Route

- Oral.
- IV (faster onset of action and stronger diuretic effect than oral)—used in urgent situations, or when oral route not possible, or when gut oedema may impede gastrointestinal absorption.

Unwanted effects

- Hypovolaemia and hypotension.
- Reduced renal perfusion and pre-renal renal impairment.
- Hypokalaemia (see following subsection on 'Potassium-sparing diuretics') and hyponatraemia.
- Hypochloraemia leading to metabolic alkalosis.

Potassium-sparing diuretics (e.g. spironolactone, amiloride)

- Weak diuretic effect when used alone, usually given in combination with loop diuretics.

Mechanism

- Either act by inhibiting aldosterone (spironolactone) or by inhibiting sodium reabsorption in the collecting tubules (amiloride).

Uses in paediatric cardiology

- Used in combination with loop diuretics to counteract hypokalaemia.
- Spironolactone is used in children with chronic heart failure as this has been shown to improve survival in adults (see p. 234).

Route

- Oral.

Unwanted effects

- Hyperkalaemia (caution when given with potassium supplements or other drugs that can increase potassium levels, e.g. ACEi).
- Gastrointestinal upset.
- Gynaecomastia.

Thiazide diuretics (e.g. bendroflumethiazide, hydrochlorothiazide) and thiazide-related diuretics (e.g. metolazone)

- Rarely used in paediatric cardiology practice.
- Weaker diuretic action than the more commonly used loop diuretics.

Mechanism

- Inhibit sodium and chloride reabsorption in the distal tubule.

Uses in paediatric cardiology

- No clear indication for use in paediatric cardiology practice.
- Metolazone specifically is used in combination with loop diuretics in chronic heart failure, where resistance to loop diuresis is thought to have occurred.
- Thiazides favoured by some neonatologists in the management of chronic lung disease.

Route

- Oral.

Unwanted effects

- Hypokalaemia.
- Hyponatraemia.

Drugs acting on the renin–angiotensin–aldosterone system

Angiotensin-converting enzyme inhibitors (e.g. captopril, enalapril, lisinopril)

Mechanism

- The renin–angiotensin–aldosterone hormone system helps regulate fluid and electrolyte balance and has a major role in controlling SVR.
- Reduced renal blood flow results in renin release, which converts angiotensinogen to angiotensin I, which is then converted to angiotensin II by angiotensin converting enzyme (ACE), mostly in the lungs.
- Angiotensin II is a potent vasoconstrictor and promotes aldosterone production, which acts on the kidney to increase sodium and water retention at the expense of potassium.
- ACEi therefore cause vasodilation and prevent the build-up of fluid that would result from aldosterone release.

Uses in paediatric cardiology

- Reduce SVR, and so increase cardiac output in impaired cardiac function (see p. 234), reduce left-to-right shunt in shunt lesions (e.g. VSD), and encourage net forward flow in AV valve regurgitation or aortic regurgitation (controversial).
- Reduce BP in systemic hypertension.

Route

- Oral.

Unwanted effects

- Hypotension.
- Renal impairment (monitor U&E).
- Cough.
- Hyperkalaemia.

Contraindications

- Bilateral renal artery stenosis.
- Pregnancy.
- Moderate to severe renal impairment.

Monitoring

- Obtain baseline BP, U&E before initiation.
- In children, therapy is usually initiated in the in-patient setting with close monitoring of BP and U&E as the dose is increased.

Key interactions

- Spironolactone: increased risk of hyperkalaemia.

Angiotensin II receptor blockers (e.g. losartan, candesartan, valsartan, irbesartan)

Mechanism

- Block the action of angiotensin II by blocking type 1 receptors found in vascular smooth muscle and the heart, so reducing vasoconstrictive effect.

Uses in paediatric cardiology

- Similar to ACEi, but less widespread use in paediatric cardiology practice.
- One specific indication is in Marfan syndrome, where losartan or irbesartan is used to reduce the rate of aortic root dilatation (as an alternative or adjunct to beta-blockers by action on the TNF pathway; see p. 184).

Route

- Oral.

Unwanted effects

- Renal impairment (caution especially in renal artery stenosis).
- Cough (although less than ACEi).
- Hypotension.
- Hyperkalaemia.

Anticoagulation and antiplatelet drugs

Vitamin K antagonists (e.g. warfarin)

- Warfarin is the most commonly used long-term oral anticoagulant (the newer direct oral anticoagulants (previously known as new or novel oral anticoagulants) have not yet been widely adopted in paediatric cardiology practice).
- The anticoagulant affect is dose dependent, occurring 24 hours after administration and persisting for 2–5 days.
- Little evidence to guide optimal use, and protocols for anticoagulation vary between paediatric cardiology centres.

Mechanism

- Competitively inhibits an enzyme that is responsible for activating vitamin K to its active form, reducing the synthesis of clotting factors II, VII, IX, and X.

Uses in paediatric cardiology

- Some prosthetic cardiac valves.
- Post Fontan completion (controversial, see p. 153).
- Cardiomyopathy with poor ventricular function (see p. 235).
- Secondary prevention of deep venous thrombosis or pulmonary embolism.
- Prevention of coronary thrombus in KD with coronary aneurysms (see p. 259).
- Some mechanical ventricular support devices.

Route

- Oral.

Unwanted effects

- Bleeding.
- Hepatoxicity (rare).

Monitoring

- Requires international normalized ratio monitoring to ensure dosage is within a safe range.
- Intended international normalized ratio range usually 2–4, depending on the indication and local guidelines.

Interactions

- Amiodarone, some antibiotics (e.g. erythromycin), antifungals, and some antiepileptics (e.g. sodium valproate) inhibit warfarin metabolism.
- Cephalosporins and iloprost enhance the effect of warfarin.
- Warfarin is contraindicated in pregnancy.

Heparin (including unfractionated heparin and fractionated low-molecular-weight heparins (e.g. dalteparin, enoxaparin))

- Not a single substance, but a family of mucopolysaccharides.
- The low-molecular-weight heparins are longer-acting and require less intensive monitoring as they have a more predictable effect.
- Unfractionated heparin used where more precise and adjustable control of anticoagulation is required.

- In urgent situations, it is usual to give a bolus of unfractionated heparin, followed by a continuous infusion.
- Unfractionated heparin requires frequent monitoring, usually of activated partial thromboplastin time, with adjustment of the infusion dose.
- Low-molecular-weight heparins do not affect the activated partial thromboplastin time and can be monitored using anti-Xa levels.

Mechanism
- Inhibits coagulation by activating antithrombin III.
- With unfractionated heparin this results in inhibition of both thrombin and factor Xa, whereas the low-molecular-weight heparins inhibit only factor Xa.

Uses in paediatric cardiology
- For 'bridging' therapy when warfarin or antiplatelet agents are indicated, but either more easily adjustable of coagulation control is required, or oral medications are not tolerated (e.g. in the immediate postoperative period).
- For anticoagulation during CPB.
- Emergency treatment of life-threatening thrombosis such as shunt blockage (see p. 315).
- Treatment of venous thrombosis.
- Prophylaxis of deep vein thrombosis and pulmonary embolism (older children/young adults).

Antiplatelet drugs (e.g. aspirin, clopidogrel, dipyridamole)

- These drugs do not reduce the overall number of circulating platelets, but rather reduce aggregation of activated platelets via a variety of mechanisms.
- Like warfarin, there is a paucity of evidence to guide use, and such use is again variable and centre specific.
- Although acting on a completely different pathway to the vitamin K antagonists and heparins, antiplatelets are sometimes used for overlapping indications, either as an alternative or an adjunct.

Mechanism
- Aspirin irreversibly inactivates the cyclo-oxygenase 1 (COX-1) enzyme involved in platelet aggregation via production of thromboxane A2.
- Dipyridamole also inhibits platelet aggregation via a number of mechanisms.
- Clopidogrel inhibits platelet aggregation via inhibition of the $P2Y_{12}$ ADP receptor.

Uses in paediatric cardiology
- To reduce incidence of thrombosis following shunt surgery (e.g. BTT shunt, Glenn shunt), or intravascular stent placement.
- Post Fontan completion, either as an alternative or adjunct to warfarin (controversial, see p. 153).
- Prosthetic heart valves, either alone or in combination with warfarin depending on the type of valve.

- Some mechanical ventricular support devices, usually in combination with warfarin and/or heparin.
- Used in high doses in treatment of acute KD, then lower doses for long-term treatment (see p. 259).

Route
- Oral (aspirin can rarely be given IV).

Unwanted effects
- Bleeding.
- Gastrointestinal ulceration (aspirin).

Vasoactive drugs

Vasoactive drugs are used to optimize cardiac output and flow. Their correct use requires an understanding of cardiovascular physiology, pharmacology, and pathophysiology. Many (but not all) operate via the adrenergic system (Table 15.1). Although the adrenergic system is complex, broadly speaking:

- Activation of α-adrenergic receptors causes peripheral vasoconstriction
- Activation of β_1-adrenergic receptors causes an increase in HR (chronotropy) and cardiac contractility (inotropy)
- Activation of β_2-adrenergic receptors causes vasodilation and bronchodilation.

Inotropes (e.g. adrenaline (epinephrine), dopamine)

- Drugs that increase contractility of the heart and so increase cardiac output.
- Infusions are commonly used in the immediate postoperative period, or in severe heart muscle disease, to provide additional support to the cardiovascular system.
- Usually given in an intensive care setting, to allow close monitoring and titration of dose to clinical effect.

Inodilators (e.g. milrinone, dobutamine)

- Drugs that produce a combination of inotropy and vasodilation.
- Milrinone is a selective phosphodiesterase inhibitor that acts to increase intracellular cAMP which mobilizes Ca^{2+}.
- Has become an essential agent in the management of children with congestive cardiac failure and low cardiac output and is also commonly used post CPB.
- Often used in combination with inotropes to produce:
  - Increase in the speed and force of myocardial contraction
  - Vasodilation
  - 'Lusitropy', a property of the diastolic relaxation of cardiac muscle.

Table 15.1 Effects of the more commonly used vasoactive drugs.

Drug	Main adrenergic effect	Effect (at moderate doses)		
		Inotropy	Chronotropy	Vasoconstriction
Adrenaline	α, β_1	+++	+++	++
Dopamine	α, β_1	+++	++	Variable
Dobutamine	β_1	+++	+	Variable
Milrinone	*	+++ **	0	− −
Noradrenaline	α	+	0	+++

+ Increase; − decrease.

* Acts via inhibition of phosphodiesterase, not adrenergic receptors.

** Also has important lusitropic effects.

- Dobutamine is a synthetic catecholamine which has inotropic and vasodilatory effects.
- Enoximone is less potent than milrinone but has similar effects and can be administered orally (IV preparation).
- Levosimendan: binds to troponin C and increases Ca^{2+} sensitivity.

Vasodilators (e.g. sodium nitroprusside)

- Potent, short-acting venous and arterial vasodilator, used to reduce SVR.
- Acts by liberation of nitric oxide.
- Cyanide is produced as a by-product.
- Prolonged usage can lead to methaemoglobinaemia.

Vasoconstrictors (e.g. noradrenaline (norepinephrine), vasopressin)

- Drugs that act on the peripheral circulation to increase SVR.

Chronotropes (e.g. isoprenaline)

- Drugs that work primarily by increasing the HR.
- May be used to buy time in children with complete heart block until a pacemaker is inserted.

Cardiac glycosides (e.g. digoxin)

- Originate from *Digitalis* spp. (foxgloves) and have been used for centuries.
- The main cardiac effects are slowing of the HR (negative chronotropic effect) and increased contractility (positive inotropic effect).
- Narrow therapeutic window, so monitoring of plasma drug levels is necessary.

Mechanism

- Inhibit myocardial Na^+/K^+ pump, ultimately increasing intracellular Ca^{2+} release from intracellular stores (positive inotropic effect).
- Also increase vagal tone, slowing AV conduction (negative chronotropic effect).

Uses in paediatric cardiology

- Some evidence for increased interstage survival in single-ventricle surgical palliation.
- Used in chronic heart failure due to heart muscle disease (see p. 234).
- Used to treat some arrhythmias (not commonly used), also used for transplacental therapy for some fetal arrhythmias.

Route

- Oral.

Unwanted effects

- Arrhythmias.
- Nausea, vomiting, and diarrhoea.

Antiarrhythmic drugs

- More details on the approach to diagnosis and treatment of paediatric arrhythmias can be found in Chapter 10.
- The most common classification scheme is that proposed by Singh and Vaughan Williams, based on the mechanism of action (Table 15.2).
- Some drugs have mechanism of action in more than one category.

A complete discussion of antiarrhythmic use in children is outside the scope of this book, some of the more commonly used drugs are discussed below.

Flecainide

Mechanism

- Class Ic antiarrhythmic (Na⁺ channel blocker).
- Slows down conduction in atria, His–Purkinje system, and ventricles.

Uses in paediatric cardiology

- Prophylaxis of accessory pathway-induced arrhythmias such as AVRT, and atrial tachycardias.

Route

- Oral, IV (rarely used).

Unwanted effects

- Relatively narrow therapeutic window, so usually need to monitor drug levels when used in children.
- Can precipitate arrhythmias.
- Dizziness.
- Visual disturbance.

Beta-blockers (e.g. propranolol, metoprolol, atenolol)

Mechanism

- Block the effects of circulating catecholamines and sympathetic nerve stimulation, by antagonizing β-adrenoreceptors.
- β_1-receptors are found more in the heart and β_2-receptors elsewhere; some beta-blockers are more specific to β_1 (e.g. atenolol) and some less so (e.g. propranolol).

Table 15.2 Vaughan Williams classification of antiarrhythmic drugs (those used more commonly in children are highlighted in bold)

Class	Example drugs
I: Na⁺ channel blockers	Ia: disopyramide, quinidine
	Ib: lidocaine, mexiletine
	Ic: **flecainide**
II: β-adrenoreceptor blockers	**Propranolol, atenolol**
III: K⁺ channel blockers	**Amiodarone**, sotalol
IV: Ca²⁺ channel blockers	Verapamil, diltiazem
Unclassified	**Digoxin, adenosine**

- Slow the firing of pacemaker cells in the sinoatrial node and hence have a negative chronotropic effect.
- Slow AVN conduction and thus have an antiarrhythmic effect.

Uses in paediatric cardiology:
- Prophylaxis of AVRT and AVNRT, and atrial tachycardia.
- Reduction of risk of ventricular arrhythmias in LQTS.
- Also used in the treatment of heart failure (see p. 234).

Route
- Oral, IV (rarely used).

Choice of agent
- Duration of action: in infants, propranolol may be preferred due to its shorter duration of action; in older children, atenolol is used.
- Bisoprolol more commonly used in adolescents/adults.

Unwanted effects
- Tiredness/fatigue.
- Vivid dreams/nightmares with lipid-soluble examples (e.g. propranolol).
- Bronchospasm (avoid in asthma).

Key interactions
- Amiodarone: increased risk of myocardial depression, AV block, and bradycardia.
- Verapamil: risk of severe hypotension.

Amiodarone
Mechanism
- Class III antiarrhythmic (K^+ channel blocker).
- Slows conduction and prolongs refractory period of sinoatrial node and AVN and prolongs refractory period in the His–Pukinje system and ventricles.

Uses in paediatric cardiology
- Wide spectrum of use including SVTs and VT.

Route
- Oral, IV (central only).

Unwanted effects
- Side effects are severe and common, which limits use.
- Rash.
- Pulmonary fibrosis.
- Thyroid abnormalities.
- Corneal deposits.

Adenosine
Mechanism
- Short-lived blockade of the AVN via the A_1 receptor.

Uses in paediatric cardiology
- To terminate SVT, or in some cases give diagnostic information.

Route
• IV.

Unwanted effects
• Chest pain and shortness of breath.
• Dizziness.

Promoting psychological adjustment and well-being

The mind–body link

Living with CHD can present a range of challenges and psychosocial stressors. Children and families often cope well, and navigating these challenges can lead to increased resilience. However, CHD increases the risk of neurodevelopmental, behavioural, emotional, social, and cognitive difficulties. Studies show that the risk of psychological difficulties is two to three times greater than in healthy peers. Such issues can impact physical health and vice versa (Fig. 16.1).

Psychological vulnerability is also increased for parents and siblings. It is important to recognize that many emotional and behavioural reactions are understandable and appropriate responses to challenging aspects of living with CHD.

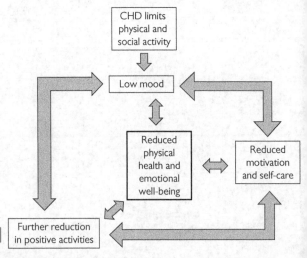

Fig. 16.1 Psychosocial stressors with CHD as a circular diagram. E.g. CHD may limit opportunities for physical and social activity → low mood → reduced motivation and interest in self-care → deterioration in physical health → further reduction in positive activities. A vicious cycle is created.

Common psychological challenges and sources of support

Diagnosis

This is a common point of psychological vulnerability, e.g. presenting uncertainty and changes to hopes about the future. This can evoke shock, disbelief, loss, grief, fear, trauma, anxiety, sadness, anger, blame, guilt, and/or loneliness.

What can help?

- Awareness of the potential impact of receiving a diagnosis.
- Consider the environment in which the diagnosis is given (e.g. private, quiet) and who the family would like present.
- Giving families additional time and space to process.
- Helping families identify coping strategies and support networks.
- Signposting to appropriate psychological support (e.g. psychologists, parent counsellors, and/or CHD charities).
- Providing children with age-appropriate explanations and supporting them to build their understanding over time.

Procedures

Anxiety is a common and understandable response to medical procedures. Anxiety is the body's natural response to threat. Many aspects of hospital can be experienced as threatening. These include genuine threats (e.g. high-risk surgery) and situations that do not pose real danger (e.g. blood tests).

Models of Cognitive Behavioural Therapy demonstrate that if perceived threat and likelihood of threat are high, anxiety is likely to be high. If perceived ability to predict, control, or cope with that threat is low, anxiety will be even greater.

Avoidance is a common response to anxiety, e.g. refusal to attend hospital/cooperate with procedures, or not wanting to talk/think about hospital. When there is no real danger, avoidance can feed anxiety by reducing opportunities to learn that situations can be coped with safely.

What can help?

- Supporting the child and family's ability to understand and predict what will happen, exercise choice and control, manage physiological symptoms of anxiety, distract from negative thoughts, and increase their repertoire of coping tools.
- Psychologists and play specialists can help minimize hospital-based anxiety (e.g. psychoeducation, hospital play, graded exposure, relaxation, distraction, cognitive behavioural therapy).
- Involving parents in psychological interventions and supporting them to recognize and manage their own anxiety as well as their child's.

Hospital admission

For parents, this may cause financial strain, feelings of being torn between caring for their child in hospital and siblings at home, and isolation from support networks. They may feel deskilled or redundant surrounded by medical expertise.

Children and young people are away from familiar routines, people, and places, they may undergo painful/invasive treatments, and see other children who are acutely unwell.

Discharge from hospital can also be stressful, as transitioning home can be daunting with parents questioning their ability to cope without a medical presence.

What can help?

- Talking to families about the emotional impact of hospitalization, related stressors, and available coping resources.
- Psychosocial ward meetings, attended by the MDT.
- Referral for additional psychosocial support, e.g. Psychologists, Parent Counsellors, Play Specialists, Music Therapists, Social Care.
- Discharge planning to consider onward referrals for psychosocial support locally if warranted.

Trauma

This refers to an event that a person witnesses or is involved in that they find very frightening or stressful. Many aspects of the medical journey can be traumatic and potentially lead to post-traumatic stress disorder.

What can help?

- Preventative, early psychological interventions helping children and families to process and make sense of their experiences.
- Education for families and healthcare teams about common reactions to trauma and when to seek professional support.
- Referral for trauma-focussed psychological intervention (e.g. cognitive behavioural therapy, eye movement desensitization and reprocessing).

Complex decision-making

Decisions about treatment may be complex and challenging for families, e.g. whether or not to undergo high-risk surgery. Elective treatments may create dilemmas between longer-term improvements and exposure to hospitalization.

What can help?

- Ensuring all perspectives, including those of the child, family, and healthcare team, are respectfully heard and considered.
- Providing age-appropriate information, to enable children/young people to make informed choices where appropriate.

- Where the child's choices cannot be actioned, conveying that their ideas are heard and valued, what needs to happen, and why.
- Working with mediation services where agreement cannot be reached between the healthcare team and family.

Adherence to treatment

Studies show that poor adherence can reduce longer-term health outcomes and increase hospital stays, anxiety, and low mood. Adherence difficulties can generate high levels of stress and conflict within families, and, in turn, high levels of anxiety and/or low mood can significantly influence adherence.

What can help?

- Effective communication between medical teams and families, ensuring obstacles to adherence for children and young people are heard and understood.
- Psychological approaches, such as behavioural techniques (e.g. reward charts) and motivational interviewing.

Exercise

Daily participation in appropriate physical activity is recommended for most CHD patients (see p. 274). Sport and exercise are important for physical, social, and motor development. Inaccurate concerns about the safety of physical activity are common among children and parents, with many mistaking normal physiological changes in response to exercise (e.g. increased HR) as cause for medical concern. This can create a vicious cycle of avoidance, anxiety, and reduced cardiovascular fitness.

Anxieties about exercise can be exacerbated by parental fears about safety. Parents may be conflicted between promoting healthy development and an overwhelming instinct to protect their child from the perceived dangers of physical exertion.

What can help?

- Exercise stress tests overseen by the medical team provide objective information about exercise capacity. This helps children and parents to learn, safely, how much exercise and activity they can participate in, thus challenging any erroneous concerns.
- Supporting parents and schools to help children recognize their limits and strengths.
- Psychological interventions for managing anxiety.

Feeling different

This may relate to physical differences (e.g. surgical scars, reduced exercise tolerance), taking medication, going to hospital, missing school, and not being able to take part in certain activities. This can create a sense of unfairness and/or isolation. Differences may be difficult for others to understand due to the lack of externally visible disability. Such experiences can generate feelings such as anger, sadness, and low self-confidence.

What can help?

• Opportunities for children and young people to explore, understand, and acknowledge differences and express and manage related challenges and emotions.
• Creating a narrative that difference is valued, supporting children to identify their strengths, and providing opportunities to meet other young people with similar experiences.

Neurodevelopmental, behavioural, and emotional difficulties

• Empirical studies demonstrate that children with CHD are at risk of developing a distinct pattern of neurodevelopmental, behavioral and emotional difficulties.
• *Neurodevelopmental* difficulties include mild cognitive impairment, impaired executive functioning, limitations in motor and core communication skills, and deficits in pragmatic language, visual construction, and visual perception.
• *Behavioural* problems include inattention, hyperactivity, impulsivity, ritualistic behaviours, sleep disturbance, and difficulties with interpersonal skills and physical activity.
• *Emotional* difficulties include anxiety, depression, and post-traumatic stress.

Exact causal mechanisms are not yet fully understood. Research hypotheses include reduced blood flow due to bypass and/or cyanosis impacting brain development and obstacles to parent–infant attachment (e.g. feeding difficulties, separation during hospital admissions, and emotional stressors impacting bonding). Physical limitations and time away from school can also limit opportunities for play, physical activity, and learning.

What can help?

• Psychological, cognitive, and neurodevelopmental screening and assessment to identify vulnerabilities/difficulties and inform interventions.
• Early psychological interventions aimed at secondary prevention of more entrenched difficulties.
• Evidence-based psychological interventions for already established difficulties.

Medically unexplained symptoms

Medically unexplained symptoms refer to persistent physical symptoms with no apparent medical cause. In the UK, medically unexplained symptoms account for a significant amount of new hospital clinic visits.

Interactions between anxiety and CHD and difficulty distinguishing between symptoms can contribute to/escalate medically unexplained symptoms. Children and parents may have underlying fears about CHD and hence be hypervigilant to physical changes. They may mistake healthy symptoms of anxiety (e.g. fast/irregular heartbeat, rapid/shallow breathing, dizziness) for signs of CHD, further adding to anxiety and hypervigilance and creating a vicious cycle.

Not understanding the cause of symptoms or thinking that others perceive symptoms as 'all in the head' or unreal can add to distress and difficulty coping with such symptoms.

What can help?

• Psychological interventions for managing anxiety and physical symptoms.

• Psychological assessment to understand interactions between physical and psychological factors, develop alternative narratives for symptoms (e.g. mind–body links), and reduce unnecessary medical testing/treatment.

• A joined-up, MDT approach to psychological intervention to enable clear and shared narratives around the nature and management of symptoms.

Multidisciplinary psychosocial care

Multidisciplinary psychosocial care

Embedding psychosocial professionals into the MDT enables a biopsychosocial approach to caring for the 'whole' child and family and reduces stigma.

- *Practioner psychologists*: assessment and management of psychological difficulties associated with living with CHD. The promotion of health behaviours and emotional well-being.
- *Paediatric neurodevelopmental and child development teams*: assessment and diagnosis of neurodevelopmental conditions, which occur more frequently as a comorbidity with CHD.
- *Neuropsychology service*: assessment of the relationship between the brain, behaviour, and learning. Assessment of cognitive difficulties which may be related to CHD. Children may have cognitive difficulties that are part of an overall diagnosis, directly related to their CHD or treatment, or as a result of the social and emotional consequences of a long-term health condition.
- *Educational psychologists*: assessment of and intervention for difficulties with learning, cognition, development, well-being, and behaviour predominately in relation to education.
- *Paediatric liaison psychiatry*: assessment and management of mental disorder, including acute mental health presentations (e.g. suicidal intent and/or plans, self-harm, psychosis, delirium) and psychiatric presentations at the interface with physical health conditions (e.g. mood symptoms due to medication or other treatments, functional symptoms).
- *Child and Adolescent Mental Health Services (CAMHS)*: Assessment and intervention of mental health difficulties (usually not primarily related to CHD).
- *Health play specialists*: support with understanding and coping with hospital visits, admissions, and treatments.
- *Occupational therapists*: assessment and interventions supporting optimal motor, social, and cognitive development.
- *Speech and language therapists*: assessment and support for developing positive, efficient, and safe oral feeding. Support of communication and language development.
- *Physiotherapists*: assessment and intervention for infants assessing neurodevelopmental motor development following prolonged hospitalization and risk of secondary neurological sequelae. In the older age group, to support both respiratory and rehabilitation recovery following surgery or prolonged hospitalization to promote independent function.
- *Chaplains*: spiritual care, and religious care as requested, to patients and families in hospital.

- *Parent counsellors*: talking therapy supporting parents/carers to process and cope with their own experiences, thoughts, and emotions, e.g. arising from the grief of actual and/or anticipated loss(es) attributable to their child's life-limiting and/or life-threatening condition.
- *Social workers*: assessment and support around the psychosocial impact of illness on families (e.g. finances, housing, childcare). Assessment and management of safeguarding concerns.
- *GP*: coordination of care and referral to local services.

Paediatric palliative care

What is paediatric palliative care?

Palliative care is an active and total approach to care from the point of diagnosis or recognition of a potentially life-limiting condition, throughout the child's life, death, and beyond.

It embraces physical, emotional, social, and spiritual elements and focuses on the enhancement of quality of life for the child or young person and support for the whole family. It includes the management of distressing symptoms, provision of short breaks, care at the end of life, and bereavement support.

Palliative care in paediatric cardiology

Advances in the treatment of CHD have resulted in an ever-growing and increasingly complex cohort of patients. These children face the possibility of multiple procedures and prolonged admissions throughout childhood, often accompanied by periods of apprehension and uncertainty for both the patients and their families.

Early integration of palliative care aims to facilitate improved symptom control and better-informed decision-making, as well as allowing families to accept, plan, and prepare for the *possibility* of death—whenever that may arise.

There are four groups of childhood conditions that may benefit from palliative care (Table 17.1). Importantly, palliative care should be considered in all *life-limiting* and *life-threatening* conditions and not simply in those children with cardiac conditions not amenable to intervention.

Specific examples of conditions that may benefit from early integration of palliative care support include:
- Children with single-ventricle conditions, such as HLHS
- Children with severe cardiomyopathy
- Children with severe PH
- Children with other comorbidities that increase the risk of cardiac interventions (such as trisomy 18)
- Children with other forms of CHD where treatment options are limited, high risk, or carry a guarded or uncertain long-term prognosis.

Table 17.1 Childhood conditions that may benefit from palliative care

Group 1	Life-threatening conditions for which curative treatment may be feasible but can fail. Palliative care may be necessary during periods of prognostic uncertainty and when treatment fails. There may be acute crises where palliative care input is required, but on reaching long-term remission or following a successful curative treatment, palliative care services are no longer needed
Group 2	Conditions where premature death is inevitable. Includes conditions requiring long periods of intensive care aimed at prolonging life and allowing participation in normal childhood activities
Group 3	Progressive conditions without curative treatment options, where treatment is exclusively palliative and may commonly extend over many years
Group 4	Irreversible but non-progressive conditions causing severe disability, leading to susceptibility to health complications and likelihood of premature death

When to involve the palliative care team

Identifying children most likely to benefit from specialist paediatric palliative care, in a timely fashion, can be challenging. This is particularly true in paediatric cardiology where the disease trajectory can be unpredictable and where recognition of the dying phase can be difficult. Referrals often occur late in the illness trajectory, with some children who could benefit not being referred at all.

For a number of conditions, it is beneficial to involve palliative care from the point of diagnosis, and this support may start antenatally. In other cases, there may be a subtle watershed moment where the child's prognosis and goals of therapy begin to change. Earlier contact with palliative care services allows patients and families to be better equipped to choose the elements of a service they wish to access and when.

'Cure-directed' and 'symptom-directed' care need not be conceptualized as mutually exclusive or alternative approaches. Although many healthcare professionals worry that involving palliative care services may be perceived by parents as 'giving up hope', research has shown that parents often do not feel this way. Planning for the future at times of great uncertainty has been shown to be comforting for both parents and children.

Types of palliative care support

Specialist consultant-led paediatric palliative care services are usually found in tertiary children's hospitals and within some children's hospices; however, palliative care does not always need to be delivered by specialist teams. Rather, it provides a structured way of delivering appropriate clinical care in a more holistic and supportive way. Core palliative care skills exist in most local community teams, among children's community nurses, and among general paediatricians and GPs.

The type of support that each individual child and family will require is likely to vary throughout the child's illness but could include the following:

Advance care planning

Paediatric advance care planning is a simple, structured way of facilitating decision-making and provides a framework for healthcare professionals, patients, and their families to document and reflect on discussions about what might happen in the future. Involving children and young people in decision-making is important to provide choice and control for the child and their family. Advance care planning is particularly useful for the increasing numbers of children with severe cardiac conditions surviving into adulthood, in whom effective transition may depend on a pre-emptive and individually tailored approach.

Symptom management

Specialist palliative care teams will be able to provide expert clinical assessment and management of complex symptoms. Children with cardiac disease can experience symptoms such as breathlessness, pain, or difficulties with feeding, and palliative care teams will be able to advise on strategies and medications to help manage these.

Coordination of care

Where possible, children should receive palliative care, including end of life care, in the place that they choose. The palliative care team can play a crucial role in helping to liaise between specialist hospital and local services to coordinate a child's care. Specialist paediatric palliative care teams are often able to support the out-of-hospital withdrawal of life-sustaining treatment if further treatment is no longer felt to be in the child's best interests.

Sibling support

Most children's hospices run programmes of activities for the siblings of children with life-limiting illnesses and/or bereaved siblings. Siblings will need support to cope with their brother's or sister's condition and death as well as the effects of their parents' or carers' grieving.

Bereavement support

Specialist psychology support during palliative care and through bereavement is available within most specialist paediatric palliative care services.

Approaching end of life discussions

Approaching end of life discussions in a routine way, close to the time of diagnosis if appropriate, and continuing this dialogue throughout the illness trajectory can help families to feel more prepared. It is important to be sensitive, honest, and realistic in these discussions with children or young people and their parents or carers. It can be helpful to discuss any uncertainties about the condition and treatment and to explore with families what is most important to them. Importantly, it is usually possible to allow space for hope to exist within these discussions (*hoping for the best*) while simultaneously discussing the possibility of death (*preparing for the worst*). These topics can feel difficult and emotionally draining for both patients and clinicians. However, approaching discussions early means that they can be kept short and revisited gradually over time. Early discussions also enable families to build an appropriate support network around them, in preparation for potential future events.

Urgent care
and emergencies

Duct-dependent congenital heart disease and the role of prostaglandin E

Background

A 'duct-dependent' cardiac lesion is one where patency of the arterial duct is necessary for survival without intervention. A continuous infusion of prostaglandin E is highly effective at preventing postnatal closure of the arterial duct and may be used to reopen a duct which has begun to constrict. Maintaining patency of the duct allows time for stabilization, diagnosis, and treatment in neonates with critical CHD.

Types of duct-dependent CHD

- Duct-dependent for *pulmonary blood flow* (i.e. critical pulmonary obstructive lesions).
- Duct-dependent for *systemic blood flow* (i.e. critical aortic obstructive lesions).
- Duct-dependent for *mixing* of oxygenated and deoxygenated blood (e.g. TGA).

Normal physiology of the arterial duct

- The arterial duct connects the pulmonary trunk to the aorta just beyond the left subclavian artery (can vary in CHD).
- The vessel wall of the duct is predominantly smooth muscle.
- Patency maintained in fetal life by low PaO_2 and endogenous prostaglandin E_2 (PGE2, produced by the placenta and the duct itself).
- The duct constricts rapidly after birth in response to increase in PaO_2 (less sensitive if premature) and rapid fall in PGE2.
- Functionally closed by 12–15 hours of age in majority of neonates.

PGE pharmacology and dosage

- Exogenous PGE rapidly relaxes ductal smooth muscle following IV administration.
- Both PGE1 (alprostadil; Prostin® VR) and PGE2 (dinoprostone; Prostin® E2) have similar efficacy and side effects.
- 80% of PGE metabolized in single pass through the pulmonary bed—requires continuous infusion.
- Local guidelines vary, but usually 5–10 ng/kg/min IV advised as starting dose.
- Administer via primed circuit to largest peripheral vein available or via umbilical catheter.
- Usually effective within minutes of administration—can be given with maintenance dextrose for faster delivery.
- Second IV line generally advised to switch infusion rapidly if primary line fails.
- In a severely unwell neonate, rates of 50–100 ng/kg/min may be considered—see local guidance.
- PGE2 can be given as a 1–2-hourly oral dose in exceptional circumstances.

Other considerations

- IV PGE can also be used to prevent unilateral isolation of a branch PA (usually left), e.g. in association with tetralogy of Fallot/pulmonary atresia (rare).
- Some lesions may still require BAS in addition to PGE if there is obstruction at atrial level.
- NSAIDs inhibit PGE release leading to constriction of the arterial duct.

Side effects of PGE

- Apnoea: usually within first hour of infusion, more common if low birth weight (<2000 g). Consider intubation if dose >15 ng/kg/min.
- Hypotension.
- Transient hypothermia.
- Fever.
- Hypoglycaemia.
- Flushing.
- Gastrointestinal bleeding/necrotizing enterocolitis.
- Seizures.
- Prolonged treatment with PGE associated with gastric outlet obstruction, peripheral oedema, and reversible cortical proliferation of the long bones.

Monitoring on PGE

- Observe respiratory effort closely—especially first hour.
- Consider fluid bolus if drop in systolic BP.
- Renal function and platelets.
- If sudden change in effect, failure of delivery (e.g. IV extravasation) is most common cause.

Hypercyanotic spells

Also known as hypoxic spells or 'tet' spells, these are seen in infants with tetralogy of Fallot (see p. 78). They are potentially life-threatening and should be treated as a matter of urgency. If spells develop, consideration should be given to expediting surgical repair, or planning an interim measure such as RVOT stenting or BTT shunt placement.

Pathophysiology

- The precipitating event may either be a drop in SVR (e.g. a warm bath), a rise in PVR (e.g. due to crying), or increased resistance of the RVOTO.
- Whether infundibular 'spasm' can occur is debated.
- All three of these events will increase the right-to-left shunt across the VSD.
- This will result in lowered systemic saturations (hypoxia), causing increased cyanosis clinically.
- Hypoxia in turn stimulates increased respiratory rate and work of breathing and increases PVR.
- This in turn increases right-to-left shunt across the VSD, and a potential vicious cycle is created.

Clinical features

- Increase respiratory rate and work of breathing.
- Irritability/crying/altered consciousness.
- Increasing cyanosis.
- Ejection systolic murmur becomes quieter or disappears.

Treatment

- Knees-to-chest position—this increases SVR and reduces systemic venous return, and so reduces right-to-left shunt.
- Morphine (usually given intramuscularly) has a depressant effect of respiration, reducing the respiratory rate and reducing distress.
- High-flow oxygen can be given to reduce PVR.
- If these measures do not work, then senior cardiology and intensive care input is required. Other options include correcting acidosis with sodium bicarbonate, sedation (e.g. ketamine), drugs such as phenylephrine to increase SVR, and beta-blockers (e.g. an infusion of esmolol).
- Beta-blockers such as propranolol can be used to try and prevent further spells by increasing SVR.

Blockage of Blalock–Taussig–Thomas shunt

A BTT shunt is inserted to increase blood flow to the lungs, either performed in isolation or as part of a more complex surgical operation (e.g. the Norwood procedure). Blockage or obstruction of the shunt is a life-threatening emergency and immediate senior help should be called, including a paediatric cardiac surgeon with theatre team.

Prevention of blockage

- IV heparin is usually given immediately postoperatively, then this can be converted to oral aspirin when tolerating feeds (sometimes other antiplatelet drugs are given in addition such as clopidogrel).
- Dehydration should be avoided in all patients with a shunt—if fasting for a procedure or not tolerating enteral fluids, IV fluids should be given.

Clinical features of blockage

- Worsening oxygen saturations.
- Change in or disappearance of continuous shunt murmur.
- Rising lactate and worsening acidosis on blood gas.

Management

- Call for help immediately, including senior cardiology, cardiac surgeon, PICU, and anaesthetics.
- Request or perform TTE, but do not delay management to wait for this.
- Give a bolus of heparin (usually 50 units/kg IV but varies by centre) followed by an infusion of heparin (e.g. 20 units/kg/hour).
- Will need PICU/anaesthetic input to perform measures to lower PVR (sedation, paralysis, optimize ventilation) and increase SVC (phenylephrine, adrenaline, noradrenaline).
- If confirmed, blocked shunt will need either urgent surgical intervention, or ECMO.

Pericardial effusion and cardiac tamponade

Pericardial effusion

The heart is surrounded by the pericardial sac, which normally contains a small amount of fluid between the outer fibrous and inner serous layers, to provide lubrication as the heart beats. This fluid can increase in volume for many reasons, this is termed a pericardial effusion.

Causes of pericardial effusion
- Infectious (most commonly viral pericarditis, but also bacterial and rarely fungal).
- Inflammatory (including autoimmune disorders).
- Post cardiac surgery.
- Trauma.
- Neoplastic.

Clinical features
- Symptoms will depend on the underlying cause and speed of accumulation.
- A pericardial friction rub is only evident when the effusion is small and disappears as more fluid accumulates.
- Examination may find muffled heart sounds.
- Effusions secondary to pericarditis may be associated with chest pain.
- Difficulty in breathing, often worse lying flat.
- Signs of cardiac tamponade (see next paragraph).

Cardiac tamponade

If the pericardial effusion is large, or it builds up quickly, the fluid can compress the heart and impede filling of the heart. This results in reduced cardiac output, and eventually cardiogenic shock. This is a clinical emergency. Tamponade requires supportive care and urgent pericardiocentesis/surgical drainage (see p. 169).

Clinical features
- Tachycardia.
- Hypotension.
- Rise in CVP/jugular venous pressure.
- Pulsus paradoxus: an exaggeration of the normal drop in systolic BP during inspiration (>10 mmHg).

Investigations
- CXR, may show enlarged cardiac silhouette.
- TTE, to look for effusion and echo signs of tamponade: diastolic collapse of RA, diastolic collapse of RV, exaggerated changes in mitral/tricuspid E-wave velocity with respiration. On spontaneous inspiration tricuspid valve flow increased and mitral valve flow decreased. If ventilated, the opposite pattern occurs. >20% variability with respiration considered significant.
- Note that the size of the pericardial effusion does not correlate with tamponade. A small, rapidly accumulating pulmonary effusion may

cause more compromise than a larger effusion which has developed chronically.

Treatment
- Call for senior cardiology help including interventionist; consider PICU involvement.
- May need emergency pericardiocentesis (see p. 169) or surgical drainage.

Normal values for paediatric ECGs

Normal values for paediatric ECGs

- When interpreting a paediatric ECG, it is important to compare to normal values appropriate for the age of the child (Tables A.1–A.5).
- The relatively thin chest wall can make some voltages higher than expected in adults, and this can lead to erroneous diagnosis of ventricular hypertrophy.
- The axes and voltages change as the child grows.

Tables A.1–A.5 were all taken from a useful paper: Rijnbeek et al. New normal limits for the paediatric electrocardiogram. Eur Heart J. 2001;22(8):702–11.

- In all the tables, the top row for each measurement is for girls, the bottom for boys.
- In Table A.1, the main value shown is the median, and the brackets show the 2nd and 98th percentiles.
- In all other tables the main value shown is the median, and the brackets show the 98th percentile.
- Bold values indicate that the values for boys and girls are significantly different.
- All amplitudes are in mV.

Table A.1 Lead-independent measurements

Measurement	0-1 months	1-3 months	3-6 months	6-12 months	1-3 years	3-5 years	5-8 years	8-12 years	12-16 years
Heart rate (beats . min−1)	160 (129, 192) 155 (136, 99)	152 (126, 187) 154 (126, 200)	134 (114, 165) 139 (122, 191)	128 (106, 194) 134 (106, 187)	119 (97, 155) 128 (95, 178)	98 (73, 123) 101 (78, 124)	88 (62, 113) 89 (68, 115)	78 (55, 101) 80 (58, 110)	73 (48, 99) 76 (54, 107)
P axis (°)	56 (13, 99) 52 (24, 80)	52 (10, 73) 48 (20, 77)	49 (−5, 70) 51 (16, 80)	49 (9, 87) 50 (14, 69)	48 (−12, 78) 47 (1, 90)	43 (−13, 69) 44 (−6, 90)	41 (−54, 72) 42 (−13, 77)	39 (−17, 76) 42 (−15, 82)	40 (−24, 76) 45 (−18, 77)
P duration (ms)	78 (64, 85) 79 (69, 106)	79 (65, 98) 78 (62, 105)	81 (64, 103) 78 (63, 106)	80 (66, 96) 80 (64, 07)	80 (63, 113) 83 (63, 104)	87 (67, 102) 84 (66, 101)	92 (73, 108) 89 (71, 107)	98 (78, 117) 94 (75, 114)	100 (82, 118) 98 (78, 122)
PR interval (ms)	99 (77, 120) 101 (91, 121)	98 (85, 120) 99 (78, 133)	106 (87, 134) 106 (84, 127)	114 (82, 141) 109 (88, 113)	118 (86, 151) 113 (78, 147)	121 (98, 152) 123 (99, 153)	129 (99, 160) 124 (92, 156)	134 (105, 174) 129 (103, 1636)	139 (107, 178) 135 (106, 176)
QRS axis (°)	97 (75, 140) 110 (63, 155)	87 (37, 138) 80 (39, 121)	66 (−6, 107) 70 (17, 108)	68 (14, 122) 67 (1, 102)	64 (−4, 118) 69 (2, 121)	70 (7, 112) 69 (3, 106)	70 (−10, 112) 74 (27, 117)	70 (−21, 114) 66 (5, 117)	65 (−9, 112) 66 (5, 101)
QRS duration (ms)	67 (50, 85) 67 (54, 79)	64 (52, 77) 63 (48, 77)	66 (54, 85) 64 (50, 78)	69 (52, 86) 64 (52, 80)	71 (54, 88) 68 (54, 85)	75 (58, 92) 71 (58, 88)	80 (63, 98) 77 (59, 95)	85 (67, 103) 82 (66, 99)	91 (78, 111) 87 (72, 106)
QTc interval (ms)	413 (378, 448) 420 (379, 462)	419 (396, 458) 424 (381, 454)	422 (391, 453) 418 (386, 448)	411 (379, 449) 414 (381, 446)	412 (383, 455) 417 (381, 447)	412 (377, 448) 415 (388, 442)	411 (371, 443) 409 (375, 449)	411 (373, 440) 410 (365, 447)	407 (362, 449) 414 (370, 457)

Table A.2 P-wave amplitudes

Lead	0-1 months	1-3 months	3-6 months	6-12 months	1-3 years	3-5 years	5-8 years	8-12 years	12-16 years
II	0.14 (0.23)	0.18 (0.32)	0.14 (0.34)	0.18 (0.48)	0.15 (0.44)	0.11 (0.26)	0.10 (0.28)	0.09 (0.24)	0.08 (0.21)
	0.09 (0.26)	0.14 (-0.32)	0.15 (0.43)	0.16 (0.44)	0.16 (0.48)	0.13 (0.27)	0.08 (0.26)	0.08 (0.21)	0.09 (0.20)
III	0.15 (0.26)	0.29 (0.50)	0.31 (0.71)	0.35 (0.79)	0.30 (0.74)	0.19 (0.46)	0.15 (0.36)	0.10 (0.28)	0.10 (0.29)
	0.18 (0.35)	0.24 (0.50)	0.28 (0.65)	0.34 (0.79)	0.31 (0.73)	0.18 (0.40)	0.16 (0.38)	0.10 (0.27)	0.10 (0.21)
aVF	0.13 (0.23)	0.20 (0-35)	0.20 (0.40)	0.22 (0.58)	0.20 (0.54)	0.14 (0.34)	0.12 (0.25)	0.09 (0.25)	0.08 (0.23)
	0.10 (0.27)	0.17 (-0.35)	0.20 (0.44)	0.23 (0.52)	0.20 (0.54)	0.12 (0.31)	0.11 (0.31)	0.08 (0.21)	0.09 (0.18)
V$_6$	0.11 (0.22)	0.16 (0.31)	0.17 (0.35)	0.20 (0.60)	0.20 (0.56)	0.15 (0.42)	0.12 (0.39)	0.12 (0.43)	0.11 (0.43)
	0.09 (0.17)	0.15 (0.37)	0.15 (0.40)	0.18 (0.39)	0.17 (0.49)	0.15 (0.42)	0.10 (0.41)	0.11 (0.34)	0.09 (**0.23**)
V$_7$	0.08 (0.13)	0.13 (0.28)	0.14 (0.32)	0.17 (0.52)	0.19 (0.46)	0.13 (0.36)	0.11 (0.30)	0.11 (0.29)	0.11 (**0.32**)
	0.08 (0.15)	0.13 (0.28)	0.13 (0.36)	0.16 (0.34)	0.17 (0.43)	0.15 (0.33)	0.09 (0.36)	0.09 (0.26)	0.09 (**0.24**)

Table A.3 Q-wave amplitudes

Lead	0-1 months	1-3 months	3-6 months	6-12 months	1-3 years	3-5 years	5-8 years	8-12 years	12-16 years
II	0.14 (0.23)	0-18 (0.32)	0.14 (0.34)	0.18 (0.48)	0.15 (0.44)	0-11 (0.26)	0.10 (0.28)	0-09 (0.24)	0.08 (0.21)
	0.09 (0.26)	0.14 (0-32)	0.15 (0.43)	0.16 (0.44)	0.16 (0.48)	0.13 (0.27)	0.08 (0.26)	0.08 (0.21)	0.09 (0.20)
III	0.15 (0.26)	0.29 (0.50)	0-31 (0.71)	0.35 (0.79)	0.30 (0.74)	0-19 (0.46)	0.15 (0.36)	0.10 (0.28)	0.10 (0.29)
	0.18 (0.35)	0-24 (0.50)	0.28 (0.65)	0.34 (0.79)	0.31 (0.73)	0.18 (0.40)	0.16 (0.38)	0-10 (0.27)	0.10 (0.21)
aVF	0.13 (0.23)	0.20 (0-35)	0.20 (0.40)	0.22 (0.58)	0.20 (0-54)	0.14 (0.34)	0.12 (0.25)	0-09 (0.25)	0.08 (0.23)
	0.10 (0.27)	0-17 (0.35)	0.20 (0.44)	0.23 (0.52)	0.20 (0.54)	0-12 (0.31)	0.11 (0.31)	0.08 (0.21)	0.09 (0.18)
V₆	0-11 (0.22)	0.16 (0.31)	0.17 (0.35)	0.20 (0.60)	0.20 (0.56)	0-15 (0.42)	0.12 (0.39)	0.12 (0.43)	0.11 (0.43)
	0.09 (0.17)	0-15 (0.37)	0.15 (0.40)	0.18 (0.39)	0.17 (0.49)	0.15 (0.42)	0.10 (0.41)	0-11 (0.34)	0.09 (**0.23**)
V₇	0.08 (0.13)	0.13 (0.28)	0.14 (0.32)	0.17 (0.52)	0.19 (0-46)	0.13 (0.36)	0.11 (0.30)	0.11 (0.29)	0.11 (**0.32**)
	0.08 (0.15)	0-13 (0.28)	0.13 (0.36)	0.16 (0.34)	0.17 (0.43)	0-15 (0.33)	0.09 (0.36)	0.09 (0.26)	0.09 (**0.24**)

Table A.4 R-wave amplitudes

Lead	0-1 months	1-3 months	3-6 months	6-12 months	1-3 years	3-5 years	5-8 years	8-12 years	12-16 years
I	0.25 **(0.45)**	0.56 (1.12)	0.80 **(1.52)**	0.82 (1.52)	0.77 (1.37)	0.63 (1.09)	**0.62 (1.16)**	0.59 (1.04)	**0.58** (1.09)
	0.31 **(0.62)**	0.55 (1.09)	0.74 **(1.26)**	0.75 (1.38)	0.68 (1.52)	0.65 (1.20)	**0.49 (1.00)**	0.54 (1.21)	**0.48** (1.02)
II	0.64 (1.28)	1.08 (1.76)	1.27 **(1.97)**	1.27 (2.09)	1.27 (2.47)	1.36 (2.20)	1.24 (2.42)	1.39 (2.23)	1.31 (2.08)
	0.70 (1.21)	1.15 (2.04)	1.33 **(2-24)**	1.35 (2.21)	1.27 (2.34)	1.38 (2.24)	1.33 (2.27)	1.32 (2.29)	1.32 (2.03)
III	0.79 (1.44)	0.76 (1.60)	0.72 **(1.50)**	0.82 **(1.65)**	0.80 (1.96)	0.94 (1.82)	0.80 (1.92)	0.89 (1.86)	0.85 (1.74)
	0.85 (1.50)	0.91 (1.82)	0.95 **(115)**	0.90 **(1.95)**	0.96 (2-00)	0.94 (1.96)	1.03 (2.09)	0.92 (1.88)	0.88 (1.66)
aVR	0.32 (0.52)	0.36 **(0.63)**	0.32 (0.58)	**0.30** (0.62)	0.21 (0.53)	0.21 **(0.48)**	0.23 **(0.51)**	**0.24 (0.49)**	**0.23 (0.46)**
	0.30 (0.61)	0.27 **(0.49)**	0.23 (0.51)	0.21 **(0.48)**	0.25 (0.48)	0.17 **(0.39)**	**0.18 (0.40)**	**0.18 (0.41)**	**0.18 (0.37)**
aVL	0.16 (0.32)	0.35 (0.66)	0.40 (1.09)	0.44 (1.04)	0.38 (0.86)	0.26 (0.58)	0.22 (0.70)	0.17 (0.52)	0.19 (0.69)
	0.18 (0.45)	**0.25** (0.69)	0.37 (0.78)	0.40 (0.92)	0.38 (1.02)	0.24 (0.70)	0.18 (0.55)	0.17 (0.69)	0.16 (0.53)
aVF	0.59 (1.36)	0.88 (1.58)	0.93 (1.70)	0.96 (1.81)	1.00 (2-20)	1.13 (1.97)	**1.00** (2.19)	1.16 (2.00)	1-06 (1.88)
	0.72 (1.26)	0.98 **(1.91)**	1.07 (1.82)	1.11 (2.04)	1.10 (2.08)	1.14 (2.06)	**1.20** (2.17)	1.09 (2.06)	1.10 (1.84)
V₃ᵣ	0.62 (1.04)	0.58 **(1.24)**	0.57 (1.20)	0.48 (1.24)	0.49 (1.06)	0.41 **(011)**	0.23 (0.63)	0.22 (0.51)	0.19 (0.54)
	0.68 (1.26)	0.55 **(0.93)**	0.49 (1.11)	0.42 (0.98)	0.43 (0.92)	0.34 **(0-64)**	0.21 (0.57)	0.19 (0.47)	0.17 (0.49)
V₁	1.10 (2.05)	1.23 (2.07)	1.32 (2.20)	1.12 (2.14)	1.08 (2.11)	0.95 **(1.78)**	0.63 (1.48)	0.54 (1.14)	**0.48** (1.18)
	1.35 (2.22)	1.17 (1.99)	1-14 (2.04)	1.01 (1.92)	1.01 (1.91)	0.77 **(1.38)**	0.55 (1.24)	0.49 (1.14)	**0.35 (1.10)**

V₂	1.83 (2.67)	1.82 (2.63)	2.08 (2.54)	1.94 (2.51)	1.82 (2.41)	1.58 (226)	1.21 **(2.22)**	**1.02** (1.90)	**0.94 (1.87)**
	1.83 (217)	1.81 (2.45)	**1.88** (2.60)	1.82 (2.36)	1.75 (2.38)	1.41 (2.25)	1.06 **(1.91)**	**0.90** (1.86)	**0.69 (1.57)**
V₄	1.80 **(2.62)**	2.30 (3.05)	2.32 (3.23)	2.27 (3.32)	2.37 (3.38)	2.42 (3.30)	2.11 (3.11)	1.86 (3.16)	117 **(316)**
	1.68 **(2.21)**	2.26 (3.26)	2.26 (3.31)	2.23 (3.09)	2.21 (3.54)	2.24 (3.38)	1.84 (3.04)	1.72 (3.23)	**1.24 (2.55)**
V₆	**1.00** (1.78)	1.55 **(2.23)**	1.65 (2.73)	1.70 (2.79)	1.79 (2.96)	1.94 (3.14)	1.97 (2.98)	**2.18** (3.24)	**2.02 (3.05)**
	0.93 (1.64)	1.51 **(2.67)**	1.60 (2.80)	1.68 (2.74)	**1.68** (2.67)	1.89 (2.91)	2.05 (3.25)	**2.00** (3.04)	**1.65 (2.52)**
V₇	0.45 (0.93)	0.90 **(1.41)**	1.01 (1.76)	1.04 (1.84)	1.14 (1.99)	1.34 (2.12)	1.26 (2.01)	1-38 (2.24)	1.41 **(2.31)**
	0.52 (0.96)	0.95 **(1.68)**	0.96 (1.80)	1.13 (1.85)	1.15 (1.86)	1.35 (2-12)	1.36 (2.31)	1.35 (2.10)	1.34 **(1.98)**

Table A.5 S-wave amplitudes

Lead	0-1 months	1-3 months	3-6 months	6-12 months	1-3 years	3-5 years	5-8 years	8-12 years	12-16 years
I	0.42 (0.71)	0.46 **(0.94)**	**0.41** (0.77)	**0.40 (0.81)**	0.27 (0.82)	0.21 (0.69)	0.22 (0.56)	**0.22** (0.50)	**0.19** (0.48)
	0.51 (1.01)	**0.35 (0.71)**	**0.32** (0.73)	**0.33 (0.73)**	0.35 (0.70)	0.20 (0.52)	0.22 (0.54)	**0-16** (0.47)	**0.13 (0.40)**
II	0.24 (0.46)	0.29 (0.55)	0.29 **(0.61)**	**0.30** (0.62)	0-25 (0.55)	**0.28 (0.58)**	**0-27 (0-64)**	**0-30 (0-63)**	0.27 **(0-63)**
	0.26 (0.53)	0.22 (0.53)	0.24 **(0.46)**	**0.23** (0.54)	0.26 (0.56)	**0.20 (0.46)**	**0.19 (0-46)**	**0-20 (0-52)**	0.22 **(0.54)**
III	0.16 **(0.28)**	0.27 (0.54)	0.30 (0.87)	0.34 (0.86)	0.30 (0-72)	0.22 (0.51)	0-21 **(0-65)**	0.19 (0.56)	0.20 (0.57)
	0.19 **(0.34)**	0-24 (0.50)	0.28 **(0-63)**	0-33 (0.77)	0.32 (0.86)	0.19 (0.54)	0.18 **(0-41)**	0-16 (0-48)	0.17 (0.61)
aVR	0.41 (0.68)	0.76 **(1.30)**	0.98 (1.47)	0.98 (1.47)	0.95 (1.63)	0.93 (1.40)	0.90 (1.51)	0.96 (1.45)	0.91 (1.39)
	0.44 (0.64)	0.81 (1.31)	0.96 (1.49)	0.97 (1.48)	0.92 (1.61)	0.95 (1.49)	0.90 (1-40)	0.91 (1-51)	0.89 (1.35)
aVL	0.47 (0-77)	0.51 (1.02)	0.44 (0.83)	0.47 (0.98)	0.40 (1.00)	0.34 (0.87)	0.33 **(0.84)**	0.28 (0.88)	028(0.94)
	0.63 **(1.17)**	0.53 (1.04)	0.46 **(0.98)**	0.52 (1.03)	0.44 (1.06)	0.33 (1.12)	0.43 **(1-02)**	0-30 (0.88)	0.28 (0.84)
aVF	0.18 **(0-27)**	0.22 (0.39)	0.23 (0.57)	0.23 (0.59)	0.23 (0.53)	**0.22** (0.52)	0-21 **(0-57)**	0-21 (0-56)	0.22 (0-54)
	0.18 **(0.38)**	0.20 (0.35)	0.20 (0.44)	0.24 (0.51)	0.24 (0-60)	0.16 (0.40)	0.16 **(0-37)**	0.17 **(045)**	0.18 (0.55)
V$_{3R}$	0.12 (0.22)	**0.24** (0.86)	0.31 (0.90)	0.34 (1.04)	0.45 (1.21)	0.53 (0.99)	0.53 (1.06)	0.60 (1.17)	0.57 (1.14)
	0.25 (0.62)	**0.35** (0.76)	0.31 (0.98)	0.34 (0.95)	0.42 (1.08)	0.50 (1.16)	0.52 (1.07)	0-55 (1.20)	0.50 (1.04)

V_1	0.74 (1.41)	0.63 (1.57)	0.69 (2.02)	0.69 (1.88)	0.95 (2.27)	1.09 (2.11)	1.15 (2.29)	1.30 (2.46)	1.30 (2.44)
	0.72 (1.48)	0.82 (1.59)	0.74 (1.64)	0.76 (1.86)	0.86 (2.13)	1.03 (2.11)	1.23 (2.49)	1.32 (2.58)	1.15 (2-05)
V_2	1.53 (2.40)	1.26 (2.54)	1.49 (2.48)	1.50 (2.78)	1.77 (2.95)	2.01 (3.08)	2.17 (3.25)	2-28 (3.44)	2.39 (3.58)
	1.47 (2-47)	1.55 (2.61)	1.47 (2-48)	1.56 (2.52)	1.70 (2-91)	1.96 (2.93)	2.17 (3.49)	2-29 (3-46)	1.87 (3.14)
V_4	1.17 (1.71)	1.11 (2.25)	1.22 (2.42)	1.25 (2.35)	1.16 (2-16)	1.25 (2.51)	1.28 (2-68)	1.31 (2-44)	1.16 (2.23)
	1.04 (1.87)	1.18 (1.87)	1.19 (2.18)	0.98 (2.04)	0-91 (2-00)	0.97 (1.75)	1.05 (2-33)	1.00 (2.28)	0.73 (1.60)
V_6	0-49 (0.77)	0.51 (1.12)	0.46 (1.25)	0.46 (1.21)	0.37 (0.91)	0.34 (0.86)	0.34 (0.89)	0-34 (0.79)	0.37 (0.85)
	0.44 (1.07)	0.39 (0-77)	0.41 (0.97)	0.31 (0.70)	0.33 (0-88)	0.30 (0.61)	0.29 (0.77)	0-27 (0.75)	0.30 (0.67)
V_7	0.18 (0.31)	0.24 (0.46)	0.22 (0.50)	0.26 (0.58)	0.22 (0-53)	0.21 (0.41)	0.17 (0.39)	0-16 (0.39)	0.20 (0.38)
	0.16 (0.37)	0.18 (0.39)	0.19 (0.43)	0.20 (0.37)	0.21 (0.48)	0.17 (0.36)	0.13 (0.40)	0.12 (0.33)	0.16 (0.34)

Index

For the benefit of digital users, indexed terms that span two pages (e.g., 52–53) may, on occasion, appear on only one of those pages.